S0-ACB-533

The New Mother Syndrome

The New Mother Syndrome

COPING WITH POSTPARTUM STRESS AND DEPRESSION

Carol Dix

Doubleday

NEW YORK LONDON TORONTO SYDNEY AUCKLAND

Published by Doubleday, a division of
Bantam Doubleday Dell Publishing Group, Inc.,
666 Fifth Avenue, New York, New York 10103

Doubleday and the portrayal of an anchor with a dolphin
are trademarks of Doubleday, a division of
Bantam Doubleday Dell Publishing Group, Inc.

Library of Congress Cataloging in Publication Data

Dix, Carol.
The new mother syndrome.

Bibliography: p. 248
1. Postpartum depression. 2. Stress (Psychology)
I. Title.
RG852.D59 1985 618.6 85-1638
ISBN 0-385-27986-8

Copyright © 1985 by Carol Dix
Manufactured in the United States of America
All rights reserved

2 4 6 8 9 7 5 3

BG

To Alice and Yasmin Eady

CONTENTS

INTRODUCTION

Here is the rather amazing story of a well-known malady that twentieth-century medicine buried. Psychiatric illness following childbearing was acknowledged by the ancient world: Hippocrates described it in the fourth century B.C. During the nineteenth century scores of very able physicians, led by L. V. Marcé in France, described postpartum symptoms and illness with great accuracy. Marcé ascribed this malady to unknown "connexions" between the organs of generation and the brain. These "connexions" were discovered in the early twentieth century—the influence of blood-borne chemicals, the hormones, on many bodily and mental activities. Further clinical studies of postpartum illness revealed unmistakable clues to its hormonal origin, and by 1935 the outlines of the endocrine system were well known. Continuing clinical studies revealed clues of the hormonal origin of these psychiatric syndromes which stuck out like quills on a porcupine. The stage was set for a breakthrough in understanding the causes of postpartum illness.

At precisely this moment, a catastrophe occurred: the medical establishment turned their backs on the historical record of postpartum illness and ignored the evidence that pointed to the endocrine system's role in "motherhood blues." Indeed, the leaders of American psychiatry mandated that the word *postpartum* and its synonyms be expunged from the nomenclature of illness. Patients with symptoms of psychiatric distress after childbearing were from that time on to be classified in hospital records as having chronic mental illnesses such as schizophrenia, "manic-depressive insanity," or "toxic-exhaustive psychosis." The assumption was that the event of childbearing had merely uncovered a latent condition. Research stood still for almost a half-century.

What caused this extraordinary denial? Malevolent intent? Antifeminism? Probably not. A curious set of circumstances led to a major error of institutional judgment—perhaps the term institutional stupidity is appropriate—and then this error was perpetuated through inertia and ignorance. The very existence of postpartum illness was denied, because no one could classify it according to the system of the day.

At the turn of the century, advances in pathology and bacteriology had led to the positive identification of the causes of many diseases. Diseases were named and classified according to the organism or agency that caused them. Several Nobel Prizes fell to the physicians who developed the new understanding and nomenclature. Psychiatrists, eager to follow suit, sought better ways to name and classify mental illness. At first they looked for a system based on *causes,* but the causes of mental illness resisted classification. Giving up, they turned to a new system based on similarity of symptoms. In the early 1930s it appeared that this might be a successful system, and enthusiasm was high. Then a "flaw" in the system was discovered: the word *postpartum* implied that the cause of the illness was some aspect of parturition.

A very distinguished psychiatrist, E. A. Strecker, who was a leader of organized psychiatry and a coauthor of the leading textbook, contrived a solution. In a paper he published with his associate, F. G. Ebaugh, he excoriated the word *postpartum* as archaic and proposed that all psychiatric illness that developed in the months after giving birth be named and classified without reference to the act of childbearing. Soon afterward, official classifications of mental illness began to emerge with *postpartum* deleted, and this is still the official position of American psychiatry.

The deed was done. The professors of psychiatry were content. Virtually no progress was made in research or treatment until the late 1970s. Then a few British psychiatrists found themselves associated with hospitals in which women with illness following childbirth were assigned to wards that treated only these patients. This specialization of care is partly a reflection of the way the British health system works and partly the result of a British predisposition to hospitalize nursing babies with their mothers when the latter are ill. First the British psychiatrists and then many physicians on the continent of Europe and in Japan began to see that they were dealing with a phenomenon that was unique, a set of syndromes that were distinct entities related to childbearing.

Professor Ian Brockington, then at Manchester, called a conference to discuss these observations, which generated worldwide enthusiasm except in the United States. An international scientific society, The Marcé Society, was organized, and it has facilitated communication between research workers all over the world. The renaissance of research on postpartum illness is underway: with new studies clarifying the complex hormonal mechanisms that are almost certainly related to postpartum psychiatric problems, and the development of two promising preventative regimes, it is likely that rational treatment for postpartum psychiatric illness is imminent.

Carol Dix has made an enormous contribution in writing *The New Mother Syndrome.* In this book, she describes the magnitude and diversity of psychiatric problems that may follow childbearing. She explores their probable causes and new possibilities for treatment. There is no doubt that physicians as well as patients will benefit from this book—indeed, that it will be required reading. With this impetus to understanding, postpartum illness should be as rare as smallpox by the end of this century.

JAMES A. HAMILTON, M.D., PH.D.
San Francisco, California

PREFACE

There was a sharp ring at my doorbell. Not expecting anyone other than the mailman, I called out to leave the package there, but the insistent ringing brought me to the door. A slender, frail young woman with deep, brooding eyes stood framed for a few seconds in the empty doorway. At first I did not even see the stroller and the perhaps five-month-old little boy in a jolly red snowsuit waiting behind her. The woman asked for me by name and I nodded. She had read my query about the "baby blues," or PPD (postpartum depression), she said, and seeing my address was so close to hers, she decided to come see me in person.

Anne-Marie was her name, and her little boy was Clayton. "I've been suffering from PPD terribly ever since he was born. I just don't know what to do," she told me. Anne-Marie had turned against food since the birth (an atypical but possible symptom of depression). She was seeing a doctor and was on some medication, but nothing seemed to shift the depression. Her husband, Ralph, was by now desperate for her to get better help. "I was so relieved to read that letter, so pleased to think postpartum depression is being taken seriously at last," she said gently.

When I finally returned to my typewriter, disturbed by the

very real evidence of PPD at my door, I found myself shaking my head again at the ridiculous situation we have let ourselves slide into. We promote the attitude that all the care and information about pregnancy and birth should be packed into the nine months *before* the baby arrives, and that no information or support should be given to mothers (or fathers) once the baby has arrived, other than tips on diapering, burping, and promoting baby's sleep.

During pregnancy, the push is toward educating the mother in the correct approach to her health and well-being while she carries the child. For labor, most of us these days attend some form of preparation class, learning about nonmedical techniques for alleviating pain and ensuring the baby's healthy and safe passage. After labor, we swaddle the baby in pink or blue, are heaped with flowers, and then are forgotten about.

As a former journalist, a ten-year veteran of freelance magazine and book writing, and then a mother, I came to the research on this book after a much milder bout with PPD than Anne-Marie was suffering. Working in London during my first pregnancy (in 1978), I had at least been made aware of PPD (in England they call it postnatal depression, PND) by an excellent television documentary that featured the famous British TV personality, Esther Rantzen.

Esther had decided to discuss openly her own terrible experience of PPD, completely to the surprise of the British public. Her honesty was striking enough to really catch the public eye, and I know she received a tremendous amount of mail from that program. Esther Rantzen at the time had her own television program, a sort of "Real People": upbeat, sharp, and witty, it was delivered on her strong personality. Esther's love for and eventual marriage to another TV personality had been covered in detail by the popular press, as it had led to a much-publicized divorce. Then, when Esther became pregnant, the news was greeted with great excitement. I remember that the day the baby was born, the tabloids ran it as a front-page headline: ESTHER'S BABY. She must have been the *last* person anyone imagined suffering depression at any time, let alone after the birth of this special baby.

Esther described an alarming array of symptoms that terrified her: she feared for her sanity. Her PPD eventually vanished of its own accord, she maintained, with the love, understanding, and support of her husband, doctor, and friends. She was able to talk about her feelings and was grateful to have discovered a doctor who not only recognized the symptoms but was able to explain their cause, which helped make recovery a swifter process.

My own mysterious bout with depression did not bring me so close to the borders of insanity, but I know now from the women I have spoken to or corresponded with that that sensation is not even unusual in the first year after childbirth. My experience was marked more by a dull feeling of joylessness, of a downward sliding, this-is-it depression. The PPD came after the birth not of my first but of my second child. Then settled in New York, I turned, like any new mother might do, to the bookstores and libraries for some explanation of this mood, only to find at most a paragraph or two in a pregnancy book, and certainly no book for the general reader that could make sense of the problem.

Obviously there should be a book for new mothers to read, one that was not laced with platitudes or determined to shift the blame back on to the woman herself. Halfway through the research I was still left wondering if I should really be taking this subject so seriously; perhaps I had invented a category of illness to defend or explain my own unacceptable behavior. I was left doubting and isolated until responses to the questionnaire I had sent out came pouring in. Then I knew my fears were unfounded. Other women did need information, did need to understand what was happening or had happened to them when, instead of greeting a much-anticipated motherhood with delight, they found themselves locked in a mood of despair.

So, before going any further, I want to offer my thanks to all the mothers who have helped me on this book. With the women I personally contacted and those who wrote to me, some three hundred mothers contributed to this book. They helped broaden the base of my approach and gave me ideas I never would have come to on my own. The letters came from all over the country: from a woman who had been eighteen on first giving birth, to a grandmother now in her fifties remembering her own suffering all too clearly.

Then there were all those women who gave me their time in personal interviews, or lengthier correspondence and phone calls: some were actually suffering depression, rocking their babies, as we talked. Understandably, no one wanted her real name printed, so I have used fictional names throughout to protect their privacy.

I would particularly like to thank these women for their generosity: Cheryl, Lucy, Monica, Sarah, Elaine, Pat, Lynne, Janine, Andrea, Lee, Jane, Suzanne, Nancy, Carol, Sue, Janet, Deidre, Alison, Linda, Robin, Laura, and Jane.

My gratitude extends particularly to Dr. James Hamilton of San Francisco, then secretary of the Marcé Society (an international association of doctors and scientists interested in PPD), for all his help, encouragement, and support during the research and writing of this book; and to the other Marcé members who have so inspired me with their enthusiasm for the promotion of the diagnosis and treatment of PPD.

Jane Honikman, of PEP (Postpartum Education for Parents) in Santa Barbara, has become a friend and colleague through our shared concern and belief in this topic, although our collaborative efforts between East and West Coast were at the mercy of time lapses and the seemingly impossible stricture of finding times, in both houses, when children were quiet or asleep and neither of us was too exhausted for a lengthy phone conversation.

My thanks, too, to Linda Lipton of the Family Resource Coalition (FRC) of Chicago, and especially to Lynne Pooley, for the work involved in compiling the remarkable and up-to-date list of parent support groups nationwide. I am grateful to Janet Spencer King and Lyn Roessler of *Mothers Today,* Vivian Cadden and Laura Mosedale of *Working Mother,* the editor of the New York *Times Book Review,* and the editor of *Birthwrites,* a publication of the Houston parent education group, all of whom printed my articles or queries seeking responses from women who felt they had undergone PPD.

There were those doctors who willingly gave of their time to talk to me about their own studies and work with the PPD or with depression. My thanks go especially to Dr. Elisabeth Herz of the George Washington University School of Medicine; Dr. Anthony Labrum of the University of Rochester Medical School; Dr. Peter Whybrow of Dartmouth Medical School; Dr. Katharina Dalton of London; Judith Klein and the Women's Psychotherapy Referral Service in Manhattan; and Dr. Adam Lewenberg of Manhattan.

The other doctor who offered me inestimable help is obstetrician Jonathan Scher, with whom I was coauthor of *Everything You Need to Know About Pregnancy in the '80s* (Dial/Doubleday 1985). And most certainly thanks to my editors, Joyce Johnson, Frances McCullough, and Anne Sweeney; and to my agent, Jane Gelfman—as women or mothers, we have been able to share many laughs on the relative "joys of motherhood," although Deborah Schneider, assistant to Jane Gelfman, was happily pregnant at the time this book was being much talked about, and all she could say was, "I don't want to know about *that!*"

On the home front—and what book by a woman with a family, can ever be written without the home being right there in the front of the picture?—I want to thank Juana Vincent and especially Jane Guenther. Their unflagging care and support of both me and the children as the baby-sitters, if that word can ever begin to describe the work of a substitute mother, gave me the time, space, and peace of mind in which to write. I want to thank Marjorie Dix for enduring the emotional crises of mothering me, and my sister, Margaret Groves, who welcomes the children into her home with much more capable arms than I can manage. Above all, I have to thank Allan Eady, my husband, without whom none of this would have been possible, and who seems to enjoy his fathering with far less conflict than I approach my mothering. Last, if never least, I must thank Alice and Yasmin Eady, without whom I would never have needed to write this book!

CAROL DIX

...th depression. My thanks go especially to Dr. Elizabeth Herz of the George Washington University School of Medicine; Dr. Anthony Labrum of the University of Rochester Medical School; Dr. Peter Whybrow of Dartmouth Medical School; Dr. Katharina Dalton of London; Judith Klein and the Women's Psychotherapy Referral Service in Manhattan; and Dr. Adam Lewenberg of Manhattan.

The other doctor who offered me inestimable help is obstetrician Jonathan Scher, with whom I was coauthor of *Everything You Need to Know About Pregnancy* (The Dial/Doubleday 1983). And, most certainly, thanks to my editors, Joyce Johnson, Frances McCullough, and Anne Sweeney, and to my agent, Jane Gelfman—as women or mothers, we have been able to share many laughs over the relative joys of motherhood. Although Deborah Schneider, assistant to Jane Gelfman, was happily pregnant at the time this book was being put in full about, and all she could say was, "I don't want to know about that."

On the home front—and what book by a woman with a family can ever be written without the home being right there in the front of the picture?—I want to thank Juana Vincent and especially Jane Greenberg. Their unflagging care and support of both me and the children as the baby-sitters, if that word ever begins to describe the role of a substitute mother, gave me the time, space, and peace of mind in which to write. I want to thank Marjorie Dix for enduring the emotional crises of motherhood with me, and my sister, Margaret Groves, who welcomed the children into her home with much more capable arms than I can manage. Above all, I have to thank Charles Taylor, my husband, without whom none of this would have been possible and who seems to enjoy his fathering with far less trouble than I appreciate my mothering. Last, but never least, I must thank Alice and [illegible] Eddy, without whom I would never have needed to write this book!

CAROL DIX

"If Rhett had understood the changes we mothers go through after having a baby, perhaps he would not have left Scarlett."

—a mother from Ohio, 1984

PART ONE

The Problem with No Name

Chapter 1

BECOMING AWARE

The mood set in after my second child was born, at about the third month. Our first baby was not yet two years old, my husband had narrowly escaped dying in an accident, my mother had just gone home, and I sat in our neighborhood playground with my adorable children feeling utterly depressed. Outsiders might have pinned the mood on my near scrape with widowhood, or on my mother's departure, but I sensed that neither was the real cause. One phrase summed it up in my mind: How had my life come to this?

I couldn't make sense of my feelings. I had wanted children, had been delighted and thrilled to meet a man I not only loved but who also wanted children. We were leading a good life. I still had vestiges of my former life as a writer (though at that point my career was suffering severe strains from the second pregnancy and my general immobility). Crazy to be feeling this way now, I said. Why didn't I feel it after our first child?

Then, I had many more reasons. New to New York, I had just left home, career, and a lifetime of friends behind in England to begin my new life in this city. I had lived through new motherhood knowing scarcely a soul, let alone having the support of close women friends, mother, or sister. Our first child, moreover, had been no dream for a new mother. She had been born screaming and seemed to continue doing so until she was nearly three years old, when finally language came to her aid and she could put her grievances into words. I hadn't been depressed then. Overwhelmed, suffering extreme culture shock from the abrupt change in lifestyle, I most certainly was, but not depressed. I had even rationalized that uprooting myself just before giving birth had been a protective device; with no former life to miss in the new land, I had been able to surge forward full of hope, optimism, enthusiasm, and a determination to be a wonderful example of new motherhood.

What I couldn't see at the time was that having the second baby had disproportionately curtailed my freedom, ruined that self-styled image of new motherhood, and consequently my whole self-image had gone awry. What I failed to see then was that I was suffering an acute identity crisis, and that was the root of this depression.

With just one baby in a Snugli (I had even refused to purchase a carriage or stroller until the baby was seven months old and her feet were dangling down by my knees, so determined was I not to feel hampered or tied down by having a baby), I had been able to cling to my sense of freedom, cling too to my former identity as a struggling writer and newly married woman who enjoyed her independence and spontaneity. It had been fun for the two of us to pack the baby in the car and go, at a moment's notice, for evening drives. It had been easy to rush into town to meet my husband after work: squeezing baby in Snugli I could still follow my whims. Having one *small* baby did not seem to have caused too many drastic changes to our life or style. But all that slid away very quickly once the second baby was with us. Then I felt well and truly saddled, as the verb so accurately describes the feeling a horse must suffer when it is tamed, harnessed, and forced to carry a burden. I had a twenty-two-month-old terrible "terrible two" and a newborn. I was no longer a free agent.

Worse than that, I felt I had been unfairly cast in a role I knew belonged to my mother and her generation, not to me. I love my mother dearly, yet I had spent most of my teenage and young adult years in a not-so-secret battle endeavoring *not* to turn into her. But here I was, after all the attempts at revolution and radical lifestyles, in effect just like her. My former identity had been a sham. I had no identity. I was a nobody.

"Oh, I'm all right," I confided to one friend who could not begin to understand what I was talking about, "but I just don't seem able to feel any *joy* in life, when I know I should."

Looking back, I can see that I had grossly underestimated the recent events in my life. My husband had barely escaped death, and I had gone through a twenty-four-hour period not knowing if he would survive, waking at 4 A.M. to feed the baby and phone the hospital. My mother had been staying with me, and although I appreciated her help, which gave me time to visit the hospital every day, she was another concern on my mind. How could I be putting her through this? Then there was the exhausting routine of feeding the baby, dashing an hour each way to the hospital, spending an hour with my husband, racing home in time to feed her again. I was breast-feeding; everyone needed me; there was nothing, but nothing, to restore my energy and spiritual levels. I felt like Samson, holding up the fragile walls of our lives.

But the crisis had passed. My husband had made a quick and miraculous recovery. We had pushed the event out of our minds. I should not have been feeling depressed.

Yet I had also overlooked another personal crisis that led to the empty "I'm a nobody" feeling. It had never occurred to me to question how my self-confidence would hold up, when my own work, so precious to me over all my adult years, had just about disappeared over the past few months. From school days on I had been a driven, success-oriented, highly determined person, and my career as a writer, choppy though such careers necessarily are, had always been very important to my sanity and self-esteem.

A dear friend, a male colleague, called me just after the birth of this second baby with his own wonderful news—his novel had been sold for one of those mammoth advances we're always hearing about. It feels so petty now, but I remember saying, "How great," in a low voice. He had achieved success, fame, and fortune overnight. I'd had a baby.

So there I was, self-esteem negligible ("My only use in this world is to feed and diaper the baby, chase and scold the two-year-old"); identity crushed ("I used to be a visible writer, now I'm an invisible mother"); feeling trapped, despondent, and consequently lethargic. I was very lucky in having a sensitive husband. I don't know to this day if he appreciated the extent of my mood, but he did make two suggestions: (1) why not give up the breast-feeding, as I was obviously exhausted, and he could take on a greater share of the nightly feedings if we bottle-fed the baby; (2) if I bottle-fed her, it would be a good idea for me to get away on my own, go back to London for a few days, while he would look after both children.

More selfless mothers out there might have said, "No, I couldn't do that to the baby." It took me only a day to think it over; by then some feeling of exhilaration was seeping back into my bloodstream. The baby took to her bottle so contentedly I felt almost guilty for keeping her on a forced ration of my own depleted milk stock.

To my mind it was an image you find in the movies: woman without sense of identity returns to former life and rediscovers who she was and is. Obviously it was simpler for me than for most mothers, as I had a convenient location where I had acted my former part. Back in London, visiting family and friends, I was "free" again. I was someone people knew and maybe even respected. What no one seemed to comprehend was who was looking after the children. What husband ever voluntarily takes on a two year old and a four month old, they seemed to be saying. Well, mine did.

The real rescue of my self came from a visit to the newspaper office in which I had worked for many years. My male colleagues had always been fun, loved to tease, and tended to refer to me by my last name—I assume because they found it amusing. That day, I had convinced myself that no one in the old department (the women I had previously worked with having moved on to other jobs by now) would remember me. I had gone first to the editor's office and begged him to take me along and introduce me. A kind, fascinating man, he looked at me strangely but agreed to escort me. I'm sure he was shier than me, for he soon vanished as the cry went up, "It's Dix!"

We all had lunch together, talking and laughing. I certainly felt like *me* again. Whether it wrought overnight change, I very much doubt. I was still elated on the plane journey home, looking forward to seeing my children and newly fired with a determination to get my career going again. It meant my husband agreeing that we would find a playgroup for the toddler and a baby-sitter for some part of the week to give me time to find work. It meant forcing myself to a strict discipline and preparing to tap into those deep wells of seemingly bottomless self-confidence the freelancer needs to face rejection and disappointment. The career did not recover magically. But just under a year later, I had work and a new book contract. I was back on the road again.

WHY WOMEN SUFFER IN SILENCE

I never told a soul I had suffered postpartum depression. Far too embarrassed, I just allowed those few months of heavy going to blend into history, as the smile returned to my face and the vigor to my step. I know I am not alone in remaining silent. Most women suffering any form of PPD not only suffer in isolation but continue to ignore or deny its existence. But that, surprisingly, is not the real reason why PPD, until very recently, has been a problem with no name.

Mothers having emotional problems? The very idea is anathema to our way of thinking. Most mothers-to-be won't even consider the possibility. Mother is "apple pie" in our society; she is security, she is steadfast when others fail; she may have a hard time juggling her many roles but she is elated at being a mother, eager to read any and every book or magazine available that will encourage, support, and improve her. Content with that "joy of motherhood" image, along with her husband, mother, and other children, she does not want to conceive of such a negative picture. Mothers cannot be depressed by motherhood, we think. They must have been prone to depression, or vulnerable to psychological disorders, before the birth.

We are in the midst of a baby boom. Everywhere we read

something about mothering, pregnancy, labor, delivery, or child-care. Having delayed their own turn for parenting, today's new mothers and fathers are coming to their task with renewed vigor, determined enthusiasm, and sometimes overpowering gratitude that they have been able to bear a child and become a family. How can they begin to accept that becoming parents might not be the fun-filled, all-inspiring event they had let themselves believe? They *know* that older mothers and fathers become parents just as well, if not better, than their younger colleagues. They *know* that working mothers can juggle roles with sufficient ease to please the child psychologists and education professionals.

The pressure is most definitely on us all. Mothers are supposed to be happy people. They are meant to adore and be adored by their children. They may be superwomen, superwives, super-moms. No one is forcing them to stay home, or to work. Yes, today's women have it all—so don't complain!

There's another side to the story. Child abuse statistics, and their accompanying sensational news stories, increase daily. Violence in the home is becoming one of the most urgent social issues. Divorce rates are catastrophic, especially among couples with children. Maternal suicide statistics are startlingly high, though never talked about.

PPD is no respecter of persons. It does not affect only the poor, the disadvantaged, the educationally or emotionally deprived. It does not care about our income level, or social class, or happiness in marriage, number of cars or homes owned. Even if we have a happy history with one or two babies, it can strike us with a new one. We are all vulnerable.

Perhaps the most unfortunate aspect of the problem is that the majority of obstetricians, psychiatrists, pediatricians, family doctors, and social workers appear to know little or nothing about this condition that can so devastate a woman's life, her family's welfare, and her children's future. Since it is not supposed to exist, women either deny its presence or suffer alone in shame and guilt.

PPD is the hormonally and biochemically induced reaction to the body's upheaval in giving birth. Research, documentation, discovery, methods of treatment, and suggested support are all available. Yet this knowledge is so widely scattered and unevenly shared among doctors at large that women still tend to blame themselves for their condition. "She is weak, dependent, unable to deal with change or lack of control, hates her mother, hates children, was obviously the depressive type or a latent schizophrenic anyway" are all common arguments used to explain mothering reactions that are viewed as not normal.

To aggravate the situation even more, there is no professional expert to deal with women after childbirth. There is no one type of doctor to turn to if you are suffering PPD. The pediatrician is the baby's doctor; once the birth is accomplished the obstetrician's job is finished. Unless suffering serious mental distress, a mother is unlikely to take herself to a psychiatrist or mental health clinic for diagnosis. This is the most crushing problem these women are faced with. There is no one to turn to.

PPD: DEFINITIONS

The PPD you might be experiencing in the quietness of your home very likely is neither catastrophic nor sensational. Your PPD may be characterized by a general depression, dullness, lethargy, and lack of joy or zest for life that has unexpectedly overtaken you since the birth of a child. Its onset could have been at any time in the first year after you gave birth.

Our biochemical makeup undergoes massive change and stress after childbirth and can, if subjected to other overloading factors —whether they are internally formed stresses of the mind or externally formed stresses of changes in lifestyle (relationships, expectations of ourselves as mothers)—lead to a temporary breakdown in the normal flow of brain chemicals that creates our natural state of mental balance. The person we used to be seems to have vanished, almost overnight. Even if we have not experienced emotional swings or depression before, we may be subject to them once we become mothers.

The two principal syndromes of PPD are determined by time of onset (number of days after childbearing) and severity. The early syndrome starts during the first three weeks and ranges from mild or moderate blues to severe psychosis. The late syndrome begins after three weeks, is mainly depressive in mood, and also ranges in severity from mild or moderate to severe. Severe cases in both syndromes usually require hospitalization.

After birth, a latent period of about three days occurs, during which there is rarely any psychological disturbance. From the third day to the fifteenth, two conditions may emerge: (1) the blues, which is a mild, short-lived syndrome; and (2) puerperal psychosis, which is very severe. Both of these share the characteristic anxiety and agitation. The blues is a temporary disturbance of mood that, apart from anxiety, will also be evidenced as restlessness, tearfulness, insomnia, and sometimes confusion. It occurs in 25 to 50 percent of mothers and often clears up in a few hours or at most a few days. It is seen as a normal sequel to childbirth.

Puerperal psychosis has the same time frame of onset, many of the same symptoms, but in addition it manifests itself as hallucinations, delusions, great agitation, marked deviation in moods, and either severe depression, mania, or changes from one to the other. The severe symptoms may necessitate hospital care within the first three weeks after birth; or, if not so extreme and urgent, the condition can merge into the depressed condition of PPD as weeks pass by.

The late-onset subsyndromes, which also come under the umbrella PPD, begin from the twentieth to the fourtieth day postpartum. The predominant mood of this form of PPD is depression. The onset is usually slow and insidious. Symptoms may include a feeling of sadness, lack of energy, feelings of futility, plus a number of physical symptoms such as chronic tiredness, delayed return of menstruation, peripheral edema usually evidenced by ankle swelling or a weight increase that is not dietary, loss of hair, severe insomnia, and a marked loss in sexual responsiveness. (These same physical symptoms can also be found when an early puerperal psychosis merges with a later depression.)

Again, there are mild and moderate examples of these late-onset depressions; there are also severe cases where mothers might be feeling suicidal or fear they will harm their babies.

The incidence of postpartum depression is twice as high as that of puerperal psychosis: two cases per three thousand deliveries of severe PPD and one case per three thousand deliveries of severe puerperal psychosis. The total, however, means about thirty-seven hundred women with serious psychiatric illnesses per year needing hospitalization in the United States alone. And if we take into consideration the 10 percent of new mothers who will suffer mild to moderate PPD, we are talking about 370,000 women each year (3,712,000 women gave birth in 1983 in the United States).

PIECES OF THE PUZZLE

Why am I saying the problem has no name when I contentedly refer to it as PPD? Let me go back a few steps to the beginning of my research. Fired by a determination to discover all I could about PPD, I began by talking to obstetricians who had made some relevant comments in the past about women after childbirth. I was introduced to one of the psychosomatic obstetrician/gynecologists in the United States, Dr. Elisabeth Herz, in Washington, D.C., who is very much involved with the problem and has been of invaluable help.[1] I also talked to psychiatrists and clinical psychologists about depression and treatments available.

But the pieces would not fit together. Something was missing. I was gathering disparate threads of information that did not add up to a whole. I seemed to be chasing two leads: it was either the hormonal argument or the psychological argument. Library catalogues did not list "postpartum depression" as a subject.

Then, in London, I interviewed pioneer gynecologist Dr. Katharina Dalton, who had previously revolutionized our knowledge of premenstrual syndrome (PMS) and who, I knew, was making a similar study of PPD.[2] Dr. Dalton suggested I contact other experts in the United States, particularly Dr. James Hamilton of San Francisco.[3] In passing, Dalton mentioned that Hamilton was secretary of the Marcé Society. I had stumbled on the very thing I had been looking for: the missing link. The Marcé Society is an international organization of obstetricians, psychiatrists, endocrinologists, scientific researchers, nurses, and social workers, all involved in work on PPD. Begun in 1980, it has produced the most encouraging work, worldwide, on causes, symptoms, and treatments of PPD.

Dr. James Hamilton, now retired (formerly associate clinical professor of psychiatry at Stanford School of Medicine), has never been one to defer his own views to the traditional or accepted attitudes of the profession; he greeted my initial telephone call with delight. "There was a flurry of interest in PPD about twenty years ago," he told me. "But since then it has died down." I went to see him in his San Francisco office and we talked away a whole day. He was as excited to meet a writer interested in a book on postpartum women as I was to meet this unique man who has for years led a campaign to get PPD on the medical and psychological maps.

WHY SO LITTLE IS KNOWN

"We formed the Marcé Society after a conference in Manchester, England, called by Professor Ian Brockington, that brought together doctors from different disciplines, for the very first time, in an effort to rectify the situation," explained Hamilton. "But it is incredible how time has stood still. Louis Victor Marcé, after whom we named the society, was a physician in mid-nineteenth-century France who knew as much about PPD as we do today."

Over a century ago, terms such as postpartum depression (and psychosis) were used by the medical profession. But, in 1926, when psychiatry was a relatively new branch of medicine and labels were being hastily sought to consolidate diseases and knowledge, a much-honored psychiatrist, E. A. Strecker, wrote that there was no such thing as postpartum depression (or psychosis), that women suffering such symptoms were really showing easily recognizable disorders such as schizophrenia, mania, depression, or other affective disorders, and that they should be treated accordingly.[4]

Such was Strecker's influence that the terms were deleted from the textbooks and from official classification. PPD is not coded for computer classification in the United States' 1980 revised DSM-III (Diagnostic and Statistical Manual of Mental Disorders) sponsored by the American Psychiatric Association; or in Britain's ICD (International Classification of Diseases). In April 1984, *JAMA*, the *Journal of the American Medical Association*, reported this omission.[5]

For the scientist intent on research on PPD, the hunt for cases becomes an endless job. All psychiatric hospital admission records of women in childbearing years have to be read through to confirm that their condition followed the birth of a child. Medical and psychiatric students are not taught about PPD. They learn, instead, the official accepted wisdom: that women—even if severely affected after childbirth—who have had no previous mental disorders are showing a latent mental disorder, and their treatment should follow the same course as any other mental patient's.

Is it any wonder women have remained silent? Not only are they ashamed, guilty, and isolated, but they are downright afraid of being classified as insane.

The nameless problem deepens that sense of isolation. Working my own way through libraries, searching for material, I concentrated my efforts at the American Medical Association's (AMA) excellent Manhattan library, looking up anything remotely relevant: "motherhood," "postpartum," "puerperal," "depression." As I came upon papers and articles, I noted their bibliographies and so tracked down much of the available material. One woman who wrote to me had similarly tried to research PPD for a graduate paper. She worked for a major pharmaceutical company and had access to their well-stocked library. She asked the librarian to run a computer search on PPD. It came up with only *one* reference, and that was a small paragraph in a medical book.

At the most recent conference of the Marcé Society, one of the leading topics of discussion was the classification problem and the desperate need for the condition, disorder, or syndrome to be categorized.[6] I have adopted the term postpartum depression and the easy-to-remember PPD. Although it is used by other writers and doctors as well, it is not yet official terminology.

THE UNITED STATES LAGS IN RESEARCH

At this first conference held in the United States, it was rather embarrassing that the Americans constituted perhaps one quarter of the attendance and an even smaller percentage of the scientific papers that were presented.

A few double specialists, in obstetrics and psychiatry, represented the handful of such well-qualified people in the United States, notably Dr. Raphael Good of the University of Texas, Galveston. The National Institute of Mental Health was represented by psychiatrist Dr. Barbara Parry. Good news was announced at the conference: Dr. Michael O'Hara, of the department of psychology at the University of Iowa, had just been awarded a major three-year grant from the NIMH to study the psychiatric and biochemical causes of PPD.

By far the strongest contingent was from Britain, whose National Health Service has been most efficient in detecting PPD in women and in treating them. Doctors from Manchester described mother and baby units attached to some psychiatric hospitals, so mothers do not have to be separated from the newborn (or its siblings) at this crucial time, and Dr. Margaret Oates described a unique experiment in Nottingham, where at-home care is provided, even for the most serious cases, by an intensive team of psychiatric nurses and doctors.

Norway, Sweden, Holland, France, Germany, Italy, and Canada were all represented at the meeting, as were doctors from Australia and New Zealand. The Japanese also were far ahead of the United States in this field. Professor Yutaka Honda, from the department of neuropsychiatry at the University of Tokyo, headed their team. Professors Bernhard Pauleikhoff from Universitats Nervenklinik, in Münster, West Germany; Ian Brockington, from Queen Elizabeth Hospital's department of psychiatry, in Birmingham, England; Merton Sandler from Queen Charlotte's Maternity Hospital, London; and noted epidemiologist Professor Ralph Paffenbarger, of Stanford University Medical Center, added weight to the scientific register.

WOMEN DOCTORS BREAK THE SILENCE

One of the most fascinating aspects of that conference, for me, was meeting a group of women psychiatrists who had originally trained as obstetricians or family doctors. I was intrigued by the success with which they had managed—as wives and mothers—to juggle the various parts of their lives to accommodate large families and careers. Three of the women had four children each, and one had six. Drs. Christine Dean, Diana Riley, and Margaret Oates from England, Dr. Judith Treadwell from New Zealand, and Dr. Ione Railton from the United States all knew the problems women encounter after childbirth, not only as professionals, but as mothers.

"I can remember only too well wanting to throw my first baby out of the window," one of them confessed. "What we have to consider is just what degree of abnormal behavior is really *normal* after birth. Every woman fantasizes and goes through some sort of unacceptable emotional changes, once she becomes a mother. I'm sure most of us have had PPD to some degree. But if you are poor, or come before a psychiatrist or social worker, those types of comments are written down as significant and as part of your diagnosis. We need to draw up some limits for what is 'normally abnormal' for new mothers."

Another said, "When I was starting in practice as a gynecologist, I was pregnant with my fourth and had three young ones at home. I'd ask the new mothers how they were doing at home. If the answer was a bland 'fine,' I'd say, 'You're lucky, mine are driving me bloody crazy!' That usually broke the ice, and then we could talk more honestly."

FUTURE OF THE PROBLEM

Although PPD occurs mainly in women who have never suffered depression before, if left untreated many of these women will continue to experience psychological problems up to four years after childbirth—and some never recover properly. Of course these cases swell the numbers of women considered mentally unwell in our society. Yet, as we will see, PPD is rapidly becoming understood, treatable, and curable by rational and effective methods.

Now is the time for public attention to turn to PPD, for research to gather momentum, for doctors of all disciplines to take the problem seriously, rather than just dismissing it as the "crazy lady" syndrome. A different generation is having babies now, a generation of women with greater expectations for themselves, with less invested in the traditional myths of motherhood. Their social role is not circumscribed by marriage and mothering. These women discuss and analyze every other aspect of their lives. If they find themselves confused when the pieces of their mothering puzzle don't fit, they will push for answers. We must stand together and attempt to shatter the myths surrounding one of society's last taboos. Motherhood is not always easy. But then neither is life.

Chapter 2

UNDERSTANDING PPD

Visiting San Francisco the first time in over a year, I phoned an old friend in great excitement—her first baby had been born on Christmas Eve and was now just six weeks old. Looking forward to seeing them both, I overlooked, even with my own understanding of what state she might be in, the reality of the situation: first-time mother with six week old in her arms.

Anne P. is thirty-six and an accomplished book editor. A beautiful woman who met and married her husband while both were still students, she has been married for seventeen years.

Her tired voice answered the ringing. "I'm sorry," I instantly apologized. "I should have realized you might be sleeping late."

"It's all right." Anne's voice lacked its usual depth and richness. "The baby woke at 2 A.M. She's usually very good. But the pattern seems to be changing."

"How are you doing?" I said hesitantly. Anne and her husband had had seventeen years of childless married life: a calm, uncluttered routine, nice jobs, two dogs to be walked, and a cabin in the country for weekends. Hardly domestic souls, she and Peter seldom cooked much at home. But she must have known, I thought defensively. She must have guessed what it would be like. She'd had us to stay on our travels, seen the struggle with my two. Surely she knew it wouldn't be easy?

Skirting the issue, as women over the centuries have done, we chatted for a while. Then I sneaked in a small laugh before saying, "Have you begun to realize yet that all you wanted was to see what it would be like to have a baby, play the game a bit? But you never appreciated the twenty-four-hour a day, seven-day a week commitment?"

"Don't worry. I've thought it already," Anne responded quickly. "There are times I wish I could send her back. Yet I don't. You know what I mean."

I most certainly did. Is there really a woman out there who has not felt some degree of the devastating change of emotions and mental outlook that follows a birth? Ambivalence is a large part of the game. Anne, in fact, was not depressed. She seemed to be coping well with the ambivalence. (A year later, I am sad to report, she and Peter were on the verge of separating.) But we can all be caught by surprise, shocked by our own reactions.

"Surely the misery I am feeling right now is a symptom of my own failure and inadequacy as woman and mother, not a definable condition experienced by many new mothers," we think.

In case you are wondering if the term postpartum depression applies to you, the after-birth blues come in all shapes, forms, and degrees. As we sit in our lonely kitchens or nurseries, we really are not alone. We are all in the same situation. It has just taken until now for us to open up and understand that these unexpected feelings are not strange.

EARLY, OR BABY, BLUES

The term "baby blues" tends to be used for a specific, temporary experience that the majority of women go through in the first few days after giving birth and that is supposedly self-limiting to the first ten days postpartum. Known throughout history as the "maternity blues," or the "three-day blues," the "weepies," and sometimes still as "milk fever" (it was associated with milk coming into the breasts on the third day), its most common aspect is uncontrollable crying. It is so common that doctors and nurses treat it as a normal part of birthing and no one gets upset —except you and your husband.

We tend to feel foolish when it takes over, for we know that we have everything to feel grateful for: we should be radiantly happy, glowing with pride and new maternal joy. And there we are crying, sometimes inconsolably. As one research paper on the early blues has shown, it can be set off by feelings of rejection; the doctor not showing proper attention, one's husband coming late to visit at the hospital, a nurse or orderly being offhand or rude; by good news, such as another birth in the family; or by a sense of inadequacy, if the milk doesn't come in properly or we have problems with breastfeeding.[7]

How common is it? Professionals agree that 80 percent of all new mothers experience some form of the symptoms: these may be the rapid fits of crying, or they can extend to sleeplessness, feeling irritable and angry, feeling hostile to the doctor, hospital, husband, and, very often, feeling confused. Up to 50 percent of new mothers have episodes of crying from the fifth to the tenth day after birth.

Most pregnancy books make some reference to the blues, with the advice that it passes very quickly and we should not be unduly concerned. "Everything will be fine when you get home," they promise us. From the women I have talked to or corresponded with, I know that most new mothers are aware of this classic early blues syndrome: indeed, they are waiting for it to happen while in the hospital.

Few of us know why it happens. Certainly even fewer know that it can attack very severely, destroying our personal vision of how we will react to being a new mother, or that even if the blues leaves us alone in the first few postpartum days, it may come on much more slowly and affect us later.

Most doctors feel that the classic early blues has a basic hormonal cause. Katharina Dalton explained that during pregnancy there is exaggerated hormonal output to hold the fetus in the uterus, create its nest, and nurture its survival. By the time a woman goes into labor, the levels of her estrogen and progesterone, for example, are fifty times higher than before a pregnancy.

The most acute hormonal change happens on the first day after delivery, when progesterone and estrogen levels plunge dramatically. Within twenty-four to thirty-six hours after childbirth the estrogen and progesterone fall from these high levels to levels that are below prepregnancy levels.

This drop in hormones can affect us in a way similar to drug withdrawal, with related symptoms. In Katharina Dalton's view, the normal adjustment a mother makes to these body changes is in fact not so much normal as *heroic*.

But many of us adjust less well. The early blues can be more disturbing than mere bouts of heavy crying for a day or two. It can leave us anxious, confused, worried about our maternal instincts. Most of the women who wrote to me had experienced something beyond a temporary, easy-to-accept weepiness.

Jenny T., 25, a secretary and a single mother, went through a euphoric pregnancy, with an incredibly successful four-hour natural delivery of a beautiful, healthy girl. She was so happy. Then, "Something got me. That 'something' was soon to be labeled the baby blues by all the hospital staff, my family, and finally, my roommate.

"My baby blues included (a) uncontrollable crying, (b) no sense of reality, (c) severe depression to the point of believing my daughter didn't need me as a mother, (d) lack of concern for the baby, (e) inability to sleep anytime, (f) lack of appetite, both sexual and for food. A male doctor said that everything I was feeling was normal. If this was normal, I wanted to be abnormal!"

Jenny was fortunate that her mother, a surgical nurse, was sympathetic and took her home to care for her. Around eight to nine months later, after her daughter started walking, Jenny began to feel all right again.

Jenny's was a typical experience. What she had gone through was not just a touch of the blues, the sort we are allowed and expected to have, but a sign of something much deeper going on.

We can begin to comprehend what Jenny was experiencing by understanding that hormonal changes are irrevocably tied to major biochemical changes within the body during pregnancy and after birth.

THE PSYCHOENDOCRINE CONNECTION

The biochemical changes may cause agitation, inability to sleep, mental confusion, or hours of uncontrollable crying not necessarily linked to a cause. The biochemistry of the body affects the nervous system: there is a more complete mind-body connection than we probably realize.

As an umbrella term, the *psychoendocrine* functioning of the body captures a complex idea. Endocrine means the hormonal system, and of course psycho refers to the mind. The words are linked to mirror the indelible tie between the two sides of our existence. We cannot have a hormonal change without a change in biochemistry and without some mental change. In our search for the root cause of the bodily and psychic upheaval, we must turn to the relatively new science of endocrinology and ongoing studies attempting to associate hormonal changes and depression.[8]

"The presentation of PPD has always been that it is a psychiatric disease," commented Katharina Dalton. "They say the woman is mentally disturbed because she has to share herself with the baby and husband. But really it is a hormonally induced state. One day we will recognize that all depressions are caused by chemical disorders and imbalances."

Hormones take their name from the Greek word meaning "to set in motion." They are the chemical messengers of the body to the brain, produced by tissues and organs. Some produce internal adjustments to the different systems of the body, some respond to external events and provoke behavioral reactions. Hormonal effects on mood and behavior have long been recognized, and current research is concentrating on how and why they work.

The hormones are secreted by the body's main glands: thyroid, parathyroid, adrenals, pancreas, and gonads. They move directly into the bloodstream to target the organs they regulate. For example, estrogen and progesterone are increased soon after a conception takes place, to protect the embryonic development in the uterus.

The brain has its own set of hormones, produced by neurons, which act as transmitters. Located in the hypothalamus, these neurohormones are directed to travel along special pathways in the brain. They, in turn, affect the output of the body's endocrine hormones. In effect, brain and body are entwined in a never-ending dance.[9]

Psychosomatic ob/gyn Dr. Elisabeth Herz helped with her own interpretation of the complex events that can lead from hormonal change to depression or mental distress in new mothers.

"In our brains we have the hypothalamus, one of the deep brain centers where physical and psychological equilibrium is constantly monitored. It regulates many involuntary functions, including sleep, body rhythms, and appetites. In the hypothalamus, neurotransmitters, which control our moods, interact with important neural hormones that stimulate all the other hormones, maintaining our systems and, usually, equilibrium.

"The hypothalamus receives constant internal input from various parts of the body via the hormones and metabolism; it also gets messages from the higher brain centers that have been exposed to external stimuli. The hypothalamus's job—influenced by a person's genetic makeup—is to balance it all out. However, if the system is overloaded—an imbalance of hormones, for example—the hypothalamus gets into a state of disequilibrium. Disorganization all around can result.

"This is why, in addition to mood changes, we also find sleep disturbances, changes in appetite, and decreased sexual desire. The regulatory system can't cope. It is a multifactoral picture, but explains why stresses that a woman could cope with at other times, when exacerbated by the internal changes, just become too much."

NATURE'S OWN TRANQUILIZERS

One main area of research today is into the actual effect of the neurohormones on the endocrine system, and vice versa. The neurohormones—dopamine, serotonin, and norepinephrine being the most common—travel along prescribed pathways in the brain, through the millions of tiny threadlike branches of brain tissue, rather like electric current moves along wires. Scientists want to discover why the current is sometimes faster and sometimes slower, how the brain hormones affect our moods, and whether medical intervention can help in cases of depression.

After childbirth, we experience major endocrine changes: the rapid drop in estrogen and progesterone, the two main hormones of pregnancy, comes within hours of delivery. There are also falls in thyroid levels (to a point lower than the prepregnant state), and a decrease in pituitary function. At the same time, we undergo massive blood loss and drop in body fluids; prolactin is increased for breast-feeding; there is sleep disturbance; and we experience other, more technical, changes, such as altered levels of adrenal steroids, free and binding corticosteroids, and gonadotrophins.

If our levels of thyroid, progesterone, estrogen, and adrenal corticoids, for example, are shooting down, the flow of norepinephrine, serotonin, and dopamine will also be reduced. The link between progesterone and mood can easily be seen, for the hormone can be used as a sedative in high doses, dulling anxiety and the agitated moods of the manic. The thyroid, too, has an obvious effect: at its highest level it makes us speedy and overanxious, and at its lowest level we become sluggish. Estrogen at peak levels makes for well-being; in decline, as at the menopause, it can lead to distress and depression.

The neural pathways along which the neuroendocrine transmitters travel, the fine branches of brain tissue, have spaces between them, which are called *synapses.* The vigor and quantity of the neurohormones at the synapses, their ability to cross the spaces, is known to be the key to mood stabilization. When the neurohormones are vigorous, we are happy and relaxed. When they are sluggish, we are dull and depressed.

Taking the neurotransmitter argument further, it is known that one vital pathway of norepinephrine crosses alongside the hypothalamus, close to what has been located as the "pleasure centers" of the brain; i.e., those areas where our relaxed, most pleasant moods are located. The norepinephrine pathway, therefore, seems to bear a direct relationship to regulating our level of euphoria or depression. The latest of the neurohormones to be singled out for such research has an even closer link with these pleasure centers. Known collectively as *endorphins* (a contraction of the words "endogenous morphinelike substances"), they are internally produced opiates that bind themselves to special receptors in the brain. If we are low on levels of endorphins we will be low on the natural opiates that make us feel good. Moreover, endorphin levels are linked to levels of all other neurohormones. Don't you wish you could go out and buy a vial of endorphins?

The idea that we can intervene with the production of the neurohormones to rebalance the basic brain chemistry if depression takes over is one of the more revolutionary and exciting new concepts. Some scientists enjoy provoking their colleagues in the psychiatric professions by saying, "In the future we will not need psychiatrists once we understand brain chemistry better." For now, however, we wait, and in waiting hope for better treatment, cures, understanding, and sympathetic doctors and other professionals. We especially hope for more discussion of PPD and how it may affect our lives.

Theories about neuroendocrinological change may not impress the women who are undergoing a surprising and unexpected bout with PPD. Examples of the early kind of blues reactions that are not covered by the "everything will be fine" comments of the pregnancy books are found in the following stories from Dianne and Kathy. Both women underwent violent reactions that left them questioning their own sanity. Both were confused and perplexed, left to grapple for reasons within their own psyches. Neither sought outside help or support. In many ways, therefore, their stories are typical and relevant to many new mothers.

Dianne and Kathy: Early Intense Reactions

I had been told of a woman going through a heavy early blues reaction. She had begun crying in the hospital and could not stop. I was nervous about meeting her, frightened of making her feel worse. But Dianne McL. was a thoughtful, reflective person. As a commercial artist and weekend painter, thirty years old, she was newly and happily married and had been thrilled to become pregnant. She had always wanted a baby and now she had a good home to offer her new family. Dianne was mature and wise. Her baby girl was beautiful, but, she said, "It all started about three days after the birth. During the pregnancy I had read several books but skimmed the few lines on the blues, never imagining it would happen to me. The books devoted so little time to the subject I was sure it was unimportant. After all, I wanted this baby so badly, I could be nothing but happy and filled with joy."

Dianne had a surprise c-section. The first few days after this, things were complicated. However, at one point she began to have hallucinations, was fearful, felt paranoid and crazy, and couldn't stop shaking.

"I remember feeling that the flowers in my room were somehow there to get me and that I didn't deserve them. They were rising up to mock me. My paranoia became so severe I was afraid that the orderlies in the hall were going to rape me in the middle of the night.

"Everything I thought caused me to cry, and all I did was cry. In the morning the friendly nurses came in, and I tried to fight back my tears. I was ashamed. I had a beautiful baby girl, just what I wanted, and she was perfect. I was able to breast-feed her, as I had wanted. Everything was perfect, but every time I looked at my baby tears would roll again down my face. Every time I looked at anything, tears would well."

Dianne later thought she found an emotional explanation for the crying within herself—she recognized a sense of loss, or separation, from her own mother (she was adopted at eighteen months). Maybe the crying was a release for all those years of pent-up feelings about losing her mother, she reasoned.

The excitement I discovered in my own research, the breakthrough I was so determined to open up, was to explain the lie, or maybe negligence would be nearer the truth, that has so affected our lives. The one thing we should all be reciting along with our Lamaze mantras is: *after birth the body undergoes hormonal and biochemical upheaval, not experienced at other times in our lives, and these changes may affect us profoundly both physically and mentally.*

The trigger that will compound these hormonal imbalances, to set off a serious emotional response, may well be found in our response to the outside world: to the enormous lifestyle changes and awareness of responsibility not held before.

Kathy S., a twenty-nine-year-old office manager with a pharmaceutical company, suffered an extreme and unexpected early PPD crisis after the birth of her son; not in the usual crying form, but with a much stronger signal. She had wanted to walk out of the hospital alone.

"I had a c-section. I came around from the operation and it began right there in the recovery room. I remember freezing with fear. I didn't want this baby! It was all a mistake. It got steadily worse. I felt so depressed and I'd lie there in bed deliberately thinking of depressing things, willfully determined to make myself feel worse."

Back at home things did not improve. "I was the worst mother you could imagine. I still wanted to run away. I fantasized taking my clothes and leaving them, my husband and son. The only strength I had in those days was not to do that."

Yet Kathy had always seen herself as a strong person. After seven years of marriage, she very much wanted and planned for a baby. She was well established in her work, and knew she would go back after a couple of months' leave. The pregnancy had been perfect. She had even carried well.

"You can imagine how horrified I was to have those feelings I least expected toward the baby. But at least I admit it. I sometimes wonder if women who crack up later in life do so because they've repressed these feelings early on, and it festers. People tried to tell me it was because of the c-section. I thought about it a great deal, but I knew otherwise. The depression miraculously lifted when Joe was six months old. I had been back at work for three months by then. I was happy to be at work. *Being a mother was the thing that really scared me.*"

LATER ONSET OF PPD

One woman had a late attack of PPD beginning eight months after the birth of her child, another at ten months. Others report onset of depression at two or maybe four months. My own case came about the third month. Until then I had been suffering the usual tiredness, the anxiety of dealing with a new baby and a toddler, and the adaptation problems of disappointment in being tied down again and wondering vaguely what I had done. The depression itself, the dark mood that I could not shift or explain, the deep questioning about my life and future, descended as if by magic at this point.

From the available pregnancy books, we learn that PPD is transitory and will soon pass. It should begin on the third day, they say, and be gone in a few days; or at worst within eight or ten weeks. That does little to help the person who begins to suffer at about the eighth or tenth week.

A PPD coming on after the second month might, we assume, be caused mostly by the social and emotional aspects of motherhood, rather than by the biochemical or hormonal forces. But there is evidence to the contrary from the description of symptoms given by women themselves. Rosie J., for example, became a single mother shortly after graduating from college and starting a career when she was twenty-two years old. Her baby was twenty-two months old when Rosie contacted me. Two months after the baby's birth, Rosie began to suffer periods of insecurity, paranoia, crying, and shaking.

"I thought I was going crazy, and so did everyone else," she said. Fortunately she read an article on PPD and realized that the symptoms were related. Rosie was prescribed a mild sedative to keep the shaking at bay. She felt it was the responsibility of her voluntarily assumed single motherhood that had so frightened her. The idealistic vision of single parenthood did not fit the reality of being young, needing to start a career, and feeling very much alone.

The blues has been defined as the agitated, distressed type of reaction, whereas the symptoms that are likely to emerge after six or seven weeks will be those of depression and inertia—the woman will be fearful, withdrawn, backward in relating to others; she will have no energy, may be constipated, and will probably find sex anathema.

The two types of symptoms, for early and late PPD, are so different from each other that doctors have traditionally viewed them as separate diseases. Yet there is an integral relationship between the two. What might begin as a mild attack of early blues may develop into the dragging form of depression, though a woman need not have had any symptoms of early blues to later develop PPD.

The hormonal imbalance that occurs in the first few days after birth may, later in the first postpartum year, lead to what Dr. Herz described as the overloaded regulatory system if the stresses and strains of adjusting to motherhood (or parenting) are so great that the individual cannot recover from the original imbalance. A late-onset PPD may well have a biochemical component, just like the traditional early blues.

TEMPORARY OR SERIOUS?

Crying her eyes out shortly after the birth of her son, a friend of mine was cautioned by her mother, "You'd better stop crying or you'll really go crazy." There is an old, and widely held, view that if we give way to the crying fits of early blues the condition will worsen rather than go away of its own accord. How can we tell if our symptoms are temporary or the beginnings of something serious that might require treatment?

Kelly M., a nurse who assumed she was quite prepared for becoming a mother, was happily married, twenty-eight years old, with a career that she felt had taught her all there was to know about pregnancy, labor, and postpartum care. Kelly's symptoms of PPD became so severe she had to receive outpatient psychiatric care and was on antidepressant medication for five months. Although cured, she still could recall the guilt and loneliness of that time, which had made her suffering harder.

Mary Ann A. had been happily married to husband David for five years, had worked as a legal secretary for ten years, and was ready and willing to have a baby at the age of twenty-nine. A good pregnancy, easy delivery, and healthy baby son were all picture perfect. Mary Ann even had a nurse's help for the first three and a half weeks back home, but still she could not sleep, could not stop crying, and began to feel she was cracking up. "At times I wanted to kill myself or the baby," she said.

Her family doctor, a psychiatrist, and a gynecologist all recognized PPD but said it was normal and would soon pass. Finally, Mary Ann's mother-in-law put her in touch with another doctor. Within hours she was referred to a different psychiatrist, who recommended that if antidepressants did not clear up her suicidal feelings within four to five days, she should be hospitalized.

Mary Ann's condition was not temporary. It needed prompt, good treatment. Back home, she took the first tablets and, maybe because the initial effects of antidepressants can be to make you *more* depressed or utterly confused, she completely broke down. At Mary Ann's request she was hospitalized that same night.

Very often, the swiftest therapy may be found in good or sympathetic care. Mary Ann's recovery began in the hospital. "I think it was the relief of knowing that someone was finally going to help," she said. Mary Ann spent ten weeks on a psychiatric ward. Her son was a year old when she was able to reduce the level of medication. Back at work, she finally realized that getting out of the house and back to her former lifestyle had helped a lot. She was one of the many victims of the ignorance surrounding postpartum women, though thankfully she found help in time.

What can we learn from her experience about the turning point from temporary to serious form of PPD? The most obvious symptoms to watch out for are suicidal feelings, a desire to hurt or kill the child, or a total inability to function, to care for yourself or for the baby. Mary Ann admitted that she had been battling alone against the stronger forces of her metabolism, trying in vain to pull inner strength, positive thinking, and social pressures to the foreground, so she would appear to be the good mother she so desperately wanted to be. Now she hopes her story can help other women, by telling them not to be afraid: "You can be treated. It will get better."

As women with more serious levels of PPD are unlikely to be reading a book of this kind, I extend my words to the husbands, mothers, or close friends of a new mother who talks of killing herself or who threatens to abuse her child. HELP HER. Do your best to find a doctor who understands and who will treat her condition sympathetically. Her negative feelings are not her fault. She is most likely incapable of helping herself. No amount of telling her to pull herself together will improve the situation; just the opposite. The new mother is undergoing, for whatever complex reasons, an extreme version of the psychoendocrine reaction. The overloaded hypothalamus has radically altered her mood.

PPD in this serious form is an acute condition that can be treated and cured, as we cure any other specific disease. In Britain and Scandinavia, where there is greater understanding of PPD and its treatment, there are now mother and baby units attached to some major psychiatric hospitals. Mothers who need admission for PPD may come with their babies, and sometimes young children, for sympathetic, nonalarmist care. These women are not filled with the fear that they are joining the ranks of the chronically insane, which tragically is so often the case in the United States.

"PPD can be very frightening if you don't know what is happening and why. I would like to help anyone who is going through it by reassuring them that it will pass, they won't be insane," said Kim S., a model housewife and mother with three children who had undergone PPD three times. The first two times Kim felt were mild, but in retrospect she could see they were becoming progressively worse. After her third baby, Kim was hospitalized, still with no understanding of what was going on.

"I really thought I was losing my sanity. I was crying all the time, panicking over nothing, my stomach would be tied up in knots, and I had acute anxiety attacks. I was just falling to pieces and why, I didn't know. It didn't make sense. I had no history of mental problems." Kim was successfully treated with antidepressants when it was finally explained to her that the tablets would rebalance her body's metabolism.

As there is very little help to judge in advance who will be affected by such a serious attack, my advice would be: rather than worry that their crying bouts are going to lead to the psychiatric wards, mothers should concentrate on making sure they understand the syndrome, what can happen and why. If they do begin to feel out of control, then together with their husbands they will have a better chance of knowing where help can be found and of how to seek proper professional care.

PMS, PPD, AND MIGRAINE

Is a PMS (premenstrual syndrome) sufferer more or less likely to become a victim of PPD? There is no direct correlation, but a woman who before giving birth has had no problem with premenstrual mood swings may discover that a case of PPD, without her realizing it, slowly develops into a characteristic PMS.

Dr. Katharina Dalton, probably the world's leading pioneer on research into premenstrual syndrome, related both PPD and PMS to progesterone deficiency. When I visited her in her London office, she explained the connection: "In the last two weeks of any menstrual cycle, after ovulation, the hormone progesterone is present in our nonpregnant bodies to help the ovulated egg nest in the uterus. Ironically, it is in those same two weeks that we might experience progesterone deficiency, if we do not naturally produce a high enough quantity. It is this deficiency that leads to the mood and physical changes associated with PMS."

As Dr. Penny Budoff mentioned in her book on menstrual cramps, traditionally women going through PMS were seen as crazies with problems relating to their own femininity.[10] But medical and psychological ideas have been forced to change.

How and why did Katharina Dalton link progesterone with PMS? "Thirty years ago, I was about to qualify in medicine, but I was suffering terrible PMS and migraine headaches. I saw a colleague, who said to me, 'Think about your progesterone levels.' I did. I gave myself an injection of naturally synthesized progesterone and it did the trick."

Dr. Dalton runs a revolutionary practice in London, where she treats women for PMS or PPD with injections or suppositories of the naturally synthesized hormone. In the United States, progesterone therapy is not used by obstetricians or psychiatrists for the relief of PPD, although progesterone clinics do exist here for treatment of PMS alone. These clinics are not recognized by the AMA and are private, for-profit agencies, so any reader should be cautious in using their services.

The American medical profession is very reluctant to lend credence to Dalton's theories, since she has not yet conducted conclusive double blind tests. As one gynecologist put it, Katharina Dalton is a charismatic woman. It might be that the women who become her patients feel so much confidence in her and are so well looked after that their symptoms vanish.

However, the link between PMS and PPD has been recognized by many women without professional help, and is certainly worthy of more research, as possible treatment for PPD sufferers could follow PMS lines. Sharon W., a full-time mother in her early twenties with two young children, seems to be typical of a certain type of PMS and PPD sufferer: trapped in a cycle of depressions.

"When I was a child, people thought I was moody and, I suppose, I've grown up to accept that I must be the moody type. I did have a peculiar early life, but even so a lot has to do with hormones. I would say 80 percent of my problem is hormonal, the other 20 percent I'll put down to me.

"I never realized I had PMS at all until my first daughter was born. Then, because PPD was so bad, I went to the gynecologist. He felt I should be able to deal with this, as an adult, and in fact I'm seeing his wife for psychotherapy. He's right, I don't want to be taking drugs all the time. But I have migraine headaches too, and I just wish there was a way I could handle it all. My husband gets crazy: it's either one thing or the other with me. I know the difference in myself if it's PMS or PPD. The PMS mood is more angry and frustrated; the PPD is crying and down."

Extending the link to migraine as well, a connection that many women will recognize as an obvious chain in our hormonal responses, Lynne S., a full-time housewife and mother for thirteen years, now holding a job as a bookkeeper, helped fit more of the pieces together. As Lynne put it, "For some reason I never connected the depressions and crying spells with PPD, until I looked back at the whole of my married life. I've spent more than half my thirteen years of marriage as a crazy woman!"

When she was twenty-one, after her first child was born, a depression began that did not go away for twelve years, until finally Lynne received treatment for the headaches that had begun when she was eleven and first menstruating. For Lynne that experience with PPD spelled complete failure as a woman. She had been the eldest of seven siblings, had helped her mother raise them, and had been the neighborhood's best baby-sitter from the time she was twelve. How could one little boy, her own son, so ruin the perfect picture?

A second child in three years did not lead to a repeat episode with PPD. Another year later, however, with two toddlers, Lynne became very depressed and nearly suicidal. She finally changed doctors, and Lynne's new gynecologist agreed to her sterilization and began to treat her for PMS.

"I still had not connected PMS and PPD with my life, until I saw a neurologist for the migraine headaches. I had begun a full-time job and could no longer afford the three or four days off work a month, caused by the migraines. But when I started to study migraine and PMS it was incredible. I was reading *my life.* There was such a sense of relief, to know that someone understood what I had been going through."

The neurologist put Lynne on an antidepressant and a vascular constrictor for the headaches. She has been on a daily 75-mg dosage of the antidepressant for two years, and unfortunately finds it impossible to lower the dose or the headaches become frequent again. With the relief of those migraine symptoms, Lynne feels in control of her life once more. She wishes doctors had understood both conditions many years before. "PMS and PPD are not just figments of women's imaginations," she wrote, "but very real ailments."

Sleep Deprivation: Barbara

It is perhaps strange that no major study has been done yet on the effect on new mothers of sleep deprivation, of broken sleep cycles that are such an obvious and intrinsic part of the postpartum period. In a recent book on psychosomatic medicine, sleep deprivation is listed as causing irritability, paranoid thinking, visual hallucinations, and episodic rages, which most of us who have been up in the night with one or more children know only too well.[11]

Broken sleep affects the rapid eye movement and deep sleep cycles, our dreaming, and our ability to store information, relax nerves, process the emotions of the day, and generally bring ourselves back together for the morning.

Broken sleep also affects the neuroendocrine system by disturbing the circadian rhythms. The term "circadian," first used in 1954, means "about a day" and refers to the day-night, light-dark, wake-sleep cycles shared by all animals. The control of our biological rhythms is involuntary and an important adaptive device enabling us to synchronize internal, biological, and behavioral processes vital to normal functioning.

Whether disturbed sleep helps create or set up the situation for depression we can only guess. Barbara B., an intelligent, educated woman who suffered an extreme case of PPD, felt that it must have been a major cause. Barbara had had a long and difficult natural childbirth, but she and husband Phil greeted the birth of their son, Nathan, with joy. During the labor Barbara had pulled leg and back muscles, so, for a long time, she was unable to sit up or walk without pain. Barbara was twenty-nine years old, happily married, living in a major city; she had enjoyed an interesting career in advertising and planned to go back to it when she was settled with the baby. She had family around her, and they were financially comfortable. Barbara was the last person she or anyone else would expect to suffer from PPD.

The exhaustion of sleeplessness, her muscle pain, the baby's needing to be fed every three hours, plus a stomach virus that she contracted, led to a chronic form of fatigue and soon to depression. She had had no real sleep for fifteen nights when symptoms began to worsen.

"At first, when I closed my eyes at night, I felt the bed whirl and saw psychedelic lights, moving geometric patterns, and the amputated heads, arms, and legs of babies. Later, when I tried to sleep, my thoughts moved so rapidly that I could not control them enough to relax. Vivid memories from my childhood flashed across as if I was watching a fast movie. I became so excited I could not lie still.

"A bizarre sense of humor exerted itself and each new problem seemed somehow astonishingly funny. I prayed, screamed, giggled, and cried. My speech became frantic and rapid. Once I started talking, I couldn't stop. Words and sentences ran together."

The mood swings were getting more pronounced, from hysteria to silent exhaustion, then crying and giggling. Once Barbara came terrifyingly close to putting Nathan down their apartment building's incinerator. Fortunately, Phil was on hand, and she thrust Nathan into his arms and asked him to take the baby away and leave her alone. Then she went into a zombielike stupor. Aware she was cracking up, Barbara herself called a psychologist for help. The psychologist, her doctor, husband, and Barbara conferred. She was put on an antipsychotic medication (Thorazine) immediately (or she would have had to be hospitalized). A live-in nurse was hired to stay with her twenty-four hours a day. Twice a week she was to see the psychologist.

Barbara began her medication, and at first progress was good, for at least she was sleeping. But she was still manic, often overdemanding, and bossy, wrote copious diary entries, and spoke for hours on the phone. At Phil's suggestion, she changed to a psychiatrist and was given a combined antidepressant-antipsychotic medication, which in her case proved very effective.

"The results were astonishing," Barbara said. "My mind stopped racing, and I found myself beginning to relax. I slept each night for ten hours, waking in the morning refreshed and hopeful. After two weeks, my basically happy personality returned." Barbara discovered Nathan waiting for her, wanting to be cuddled and loved. The psychiatrist announced that she no longer needed to be a patient and could stop taking the medication, warning her that she must get enough sleep and not tire herself out. Barbara couldn't believe it all happened to her, which is why she was intrigued by the question of sleep deprivation and its effects on new mothers.

In trying to understand the complex picture of PPD, we have first to overcome years, if not centuries, of misinformation, negligence, and psychological dumping on women of what is now obviously a biochemically induced syndrome (or syndromes because there is more than one manifestation of PPD). But you will still find doctors, psychiatrists, and scientists arguing over the relative importance of the biochemical or psychogenic makeup of the emotional condition the new mother finds herself in. So let us turn to a closer examination of how PPD has been regarded in history and the major breakthroughs in research and treatment that are currently underway.

Chapter 3

PPD: PAST, PRESENT, AND FUTURE

The first description of postpartum mental illness comes from the fourth century B.C., by Hippocrates, in the *Third Book of Epidemics.*[12] Hippocrates cited the case of a woman who gave birth to twins, experienced severe insomnia and restlessness on the sixth day postpartum, became delirious on the eleventh day and then comatose, and she died on the seventeenth day. Hippocrates offered two hypotheses for the cause of her postpartum mental illness: (1) that lochial discharge, when suppressed, could be carried toward the head and result in agitation (the *lochia* being the blood discharge following delivery); and (2) that "when blood collects at the breasts of a woman, it indicates madness." His hypotheses became the medical dogma for the condition for the next two thousand years.

The nineteenth century saw a revival of interest in postpartum mental disorders. The French doctor Esquirol published a two-volume *Des Maladies Mentales* in 1838, with a forty-three-page discussion of postpartum women. He based his discussion on the ninety-two cases he had observed, noting that postpartum illness could occur in a variety of syndromes and suggesting that several causal factors might be responsible: heredity, "extreme susceptibility," previous attacks after childbirth, emotional instability, and traumatic events.

The methods of treatment recommended by Esquirol included careful nursing, tepid baths, and purgatives. He also believed that the incidence of such disorders was greater than statistics indicated because a large number of mild to moderate cases were cared for at home by relatives and were never recorded (a situation that continues today).

Early in the nineteenth century it became customary to separate events and diseases that occurred after childbirth into two categories: (1) "puerperal" if it happened within six weeks of childbirth, and (2) "lactational" if it came on after six weeks. For decades, psychiatrists used to separate the two groups rigidly on this six-week baseline.

Treatment for postpartum women in nineteenth-century America used to be baths at a temperature of 94 to 98° F and large doses of opium. In England, at the same time, postpartum women were being treated by bloodletting, restraint (they were tied to the bed), or with opium and Indian hemp.

A courtroom battle at the Lent assizes in Essex, England, in 1848 stimulated much public and medical interest in postpartum problems and led to sensationalized news stories of infanticide and postpartum conditions for many years. The case was of a woman accused of murdering her child by slitting its throat. Her doctor testified that she had been suffering from puerperal mania and was not guilty on grounds of insanity. The lord chief justice criticized the doctor's testimony as rash and carelessly given, but the jury disregarded his directives and returned a verdict of not guilty because of insanity. The lord chief justice then came in for widespread criticism, as his own *father* had been a famous obstetrician who had written on the hazards of suicide and infanticide after childbirth.

The most outstanding contribution to the literature of such problems was Marcé's book, *Traité de la Folie des Femmes Enceintes*, published in 1858. It is still the *only* comprehensive book in the world literature on this subject. The Marcé Society took its name in memory of this brilliant young French doctor. Louis Victor Marcé was born in 1828 and, as a medical student in

Nantes, soon built up a brilliant reputation in the psychiatric field of medicine. In need of money to support a new wife, after completing his medical training he accepted a post in the mental hospital at Ivry-sur-Seine, which had been founded by the famous Esquirol. Marcé was encouraged to continue the observations on mental illness after childbirth that had been begun by Esquirol. The young doctor was thirty years old when his book was published.

Four years later he published a 672-page book, *Traité Pratique des Maladies Mentales.* Just two years later, at the age of thirty-six, he was dead. Since his death, medical science has lagged behind those Victorian pioneers in research and interest, due largely to internal squabbles between the professions of obstetrics and psychiatry.

Marcé had been struck by the tandem march of psychological syndromes and physical changes that follows childbirth. He had believed in a connection between reproduction and the brain, suspecting there was a connection between abnormal psychology and abnormal behavior. He used the term *sympathie morbide.* Marcé's conclusions foresaw the birth of the science of endocrinology.

Since the nineteenth-century spurt of interest, however, progress has been decidedly slow. When I met Dr. Hamilton in his busy San Francisco office he apologized for acting like a television evangelist who gets his audience by the sleeve and won't let go till they are also believers. But this remarkable man has carried out a campaign for the past twenty years to have PPD accepted as a disease, to have the classification changed.

Hamilton's *Postpartum Psychiatric Problems,* written more than twenty years ago, dealt with many cases in his own practice. He genuinely had hoped that the impact of the book would result in PPD's reclassification. "But by 1975, when I realized that I had not dented the establishment one iota, I embarked on an eighteen-month campaign to reclassify the condition. I cajoled, cried, threatened, worked on committees, and still made no progress." Since the formation of the Marcé Society, however, Hamilton has joined with several other internationally renowned doctors and psychiatrists, and the results are at last encouraging.

The conference held in Manchester, England, in June 1980 brought together a disparate group of people who were impressed over the course of 48 hours, by the evidence of an explosive growth of information that was developing in many professional areas besides psychiatry: obstetrics, endocrinology, nursing, social services, and others. At the end of the conference, a group of doctors came together and agreed to work toward better communication. The founding members of the Marcé Society were Professor Ian Brockington, now of Queen Elizabeth Hospital, Birmingham, England; Professor R. E. Kendell, of the Department of Psychiatry, Edinburgh Hospital, Edinburgh, Scotland; Dr. Channi Kumar, of the Institute of Psychiatry, London, England; Professor Ralph Paffenbarger, of the Department of Epidemiology, Stanford School of Medicine, Stanford, California; Dr. James Hamilton, of San Francisco, California; and Professor George Winokur, of the Department of Psychiatry, University of Iowa.

Nancy: Problems of Misdiagnosis

At the 1984 conference of the Marcé Society, it was agreed: "Step one is to acknowledge the unique features of postpartum illness by stopping its enforced classification with chronic psychiatric illness and by giving it the identity of its own name, or names. This is a primary goal of the Marcé Society."

In the Diagnostic and Statistical Manual (DSM-III) (published by the American Psychiatric Association), the reference for postpartum mental disorders reads: "Postpartum psychosis. See Schizophrenic disorder, Brief reactive psychosis, Major affective disorders, Organic brain syndrome."

While we are considering the effects of this lack of classification of PPD as a mental disorder related specifically to childbirth, we should look at a case and appreciate just how the lack of understanding affects the individual and the family.

Like any woman's story, if we dig deep enough, Nancy E.'s example has much of an individual nature that led to her own overloaded circuits. A former elementary school teacher turned administrative assistant in her husband's business, mother to an eight year old, stepmother to four other children, and new mother to a four-month-old baby, Nancy's swift decline into severe PPD began a couple of months after her triumphant return home from the hospital with baby Val, who, she dreamed, would finally complete the family she loved and intended to keep so happy.

But this second baby was not the angel her elder sister had been. Colic, screaming, sleepless night after sleepless night, and lack of support from her pediatrician, friends, or family finally led Nancy to collapse on the bedroom floor at six in the morning, begging her husband to help her.

She was rushed to the hospital where she was sedated, and sleep did, indeed, seem to offer the magic cure. (For Val, too, who took a bottle and fell gratefully to sleep). The symptoms of PPD proper had not even then begun to appear. Only after she returned home, maintained Val on a routine, and seemingly was getting herself back to normal life did Nancy show the disturbing symptoms. "I began to have severe anxiety attacks. I really thought I was losing my mind. I would sit talking to friends feeling completely distanced from them, and from the baby, wondering if they could see I was crazy."

The danger signals that Nancy overlooked were her fleeting thoughts of suicide, her chronic guilt for being this way, and her complete lack of self-worth.

Her husband, David, took Nancy to see a psychiatrist. Now feeling ashamed as well as guilty, at first she was relieved to learn that her condition was depression. On antidepressant medication Nancy began to feel more like her old self in a week or two. But the psychiatrist's diagnosis of her condition as melancholia—in itself an archaic misnomer—which might last for several years (with periods of remission), burdened her with guilt, shame, and revulsion at the thought of her change in mental well-being. How had this come to pass when she had been such a happy, contented woman?

When Nancy and David later had to change their medical coverage, she found that one company refused to offer her benefits because of this history of "mental disease." As far as the psychological profession and the insurance companies were concerned, Nancy had joined the ranks of the chronically insane.

When Nancy first contacted me it was with great relief that she had finally read something about PPD. "Until I saw your article, by accident, I had never heard of PPD. I had vaguely heard of the baby blues, but I had no idea that there was a condition, quite common, that can be treated with short-term therapy and that does not mean we are permanently ill. I'm the type who reads everything on childcare possible. Without your article, I would still be worrying that I was seriously mentally ill."

Nancy had to continue with antidepressant medication until slowly her mood lifted. Val turned into an angel, and Nancy returned to part-time work with her husband, two days a week. She found that getting back into work, freeing herself from the house and childcare routine, helped restore that vulnerable balance we call mental well-being. Like many women, she has had to learn a more realistic view of motherhood, to adapt some of her childlike fantasies of herself as a mother to herself as an adult in today's world.

CURRENT DIRECTIONS

The three main arguments in today's attitudes toward PPD remain that (1) it is not linked at all with childbirth but merely is symptomatic of latent psychological vulnerability in the woman; (2) the psychological stress of becoming a mother is the sole cause of PPD; (3) the act of childbirth sets off neuroendocrinological changes not otherwise experienced in daily life.

The psychological aspects of mothering that might help trigger onset of PPD are discussed in Part Two. For now, I want to concentrate on the various avenues of thought that scientists and doctors are currently pursuing in their search for the biochemical cause and treatment of PPD.

Let us look at the effect of one important pregnancy hormone: *thyroid.* Both the thyroid gland and the pituitary increase and enlarge during pregnancy. After childbirth, the level of thyroid slowly decreases in the following weeks to a level lower than before pregnancy, and it remains low for a year or more. The effects of a low thyroid level do not show up in those cases of agitated early blues, but in the PPDs that begin two to four weeks after birth, that often continue for the whole of the first year of the child's life. Although thyroid deprivation (hypothyroidism) has not been proven as a cause of mental disorder after childbirth, symptoms certainly seem related. Hypothyroidism leaves a victim mentally slow, lethargic, melancholy, having headaches, and feeling the cold. A mother so affected also feels no joy or happiness, has difficulty in thinking, has a poor memory and slow speech, and is highly emotional. She might even suffer amenorrhea (no periods) or find that her hair is falling out. All are symptoms of the late type of PPD that characteristically develops four weeks or so after childbirth.

Dr. Hamilton came to the thyroid connection when a woman was referred to him who had been given electric shock treatments (ECT) at a nearby hospital, deemed cured, and allowed to go home. She had previously been released from the prestigious Mayo Clinic after treatment for severe PPD. Within days of discharge she had fallen to pieces and tried to commit suicide. Her desperate family turned to Hamilton for help.

Hamilton ran every possible test on the woman. He found only a thyroid deficiency, so he treated her with thyroxine. The cure was striking in its speed and thoroughness. As Hamilton said, "You see a woman whose feet are swollen, who has slowness of speech, is very fatigued, her hair is falling out, and she has no interest in sex; then you find a thyroid deficiency, give her thyroxine, and she feels good; it does not take a genius to realize the thyroid medication was good not only for the swollen feet, but for her mood. Many doctors have noticed and connected it. But as yet it has not been accepted as a valid treatment for PPD."

Thyroid has been connected with mental disorders, even in the public mind, since the 1937 publication of A. J. Cronin's novel *The Citadel.* Watching the recent dramatization of the novel on PBS, I was struck by the appalling circumstances that had led victims of "myxedema" to be straight-jacketed and committed for life to insane asylums, when a short course of thyroid medication cured them completely.

THE DRAMATIC EFFECTS OF THYROID

Pamela D., a woman in her mid-thirties, described her own particular experience of thyroid irregularity, which she became aware of after surgery for a benign cyst on the thyroid gland. The symptoms were not directly related to giving birth (though she had had two children in the past four years), but serve to show the dramatic effect thyroid imbalance can have on the body and the mind.

"I had been suffering anxiety, insomnia, loss of weight, huge appetite, nervous hands and general speediness, and had almost taken myself to a psychiatrist, when I discovered the lump in my neck myself. The effect of the cyst was obviously to increase thyroid production, although according to the blood tests my thyroid was not hyperactive. However, the most dramatic effects of thyroid changes came when I returned home following surgery to remove the cyst and one lobe of the thyroid gland. I had been assured that tests showed my thyroid function had immediately returned to normal and I was showing no ill-effects of the surgery (and the lump had been benign so I had no cause for fear). But that first night home, I experienced the most awful wakeful nightmares that filled me with terror.

"I was convinced the room was filled with an electrical charge, that I was an evil spirit, that the furniture was hostile to me. I fled downstairs, shaking, and tried to pull myself together. I had never experienced hallucinations or been delirious at any time in my life, and was consequently horrified by the strength of those feelings. I now understand and sympathize more with people who go through mental illness. The feelings are out of your control. It was as though something was taking me over from within."

Marsha H., a TV producer, was also able to point the finger at thyroid. Apart from early problems with breast-feeding, and her age (she was over thirty-five and that made her feel inadequate as a new mother), Marsha adjusted quickly to the sheer delight and joy in baby Jason, whom both she and her journalist husband, Bob, adored. Everything should have been fine. Marsha was working just one or two days a week, easing herself back into her career. Even that proved too much. Fatigue, despair, uncontrollable agitation, and mood swings drove her to stagger to the family doctor, when Jason was just five weeks old. She collapsed in floods of tears and rage. Marsha had no strength left. "I had become impossible to live with, full of tension, generally unable to cope with my stress. I was snapping and shouting at Bob, which is not really my nature, and certainly not something I was used to doing with him; he is such a kind and supportive man. Consequently I was getting more and more depressed—at myself."

At first the doctor gave Marsha tranquilizers to control her mood, but they only made her more tired and less able to cope. When she turned to another doctor, who ran some blood tests, it was discovered by accident that Marsha had an almost nonfunctioning thyroid. Marsha had told the doctor that hypothyroidism ran in her family, as it had affected both her mother and sister, but the doctor did not think there was anything in it until he ran the tests. Marsha was then treated with thyroxine. Although she had no overnight cure, her progress was slow and sure. Her case was unusual in that her thyroid deficit was so low as to be glaringly obvious. Unfortunately for research into thyroid deficiency and PPD, convincing results are hard to come by. Hamilton reacted severely to the prospect of running double blind tests on postpartum women, especially if they were suicidal or severely depressed, because offering a placebo instead of the thyroxine to these women would be downright cruel.

Further complicating the matter, as psychiatrist Junich Nomura and thyroidologist Nobuyuki Amino, both of Japan, have reported, an early agitated case of severe PPD may result from abnormally *high* levels of thyroxine in the blood.[13] As research at this level is very new, psychiatrists would have to work in tandem with good endocrinologists when treating women with thyroid therapy.

ADRENAL CORTICOIDS: AN ANSWER?

The 1984 conference of the Marcé Society revealed many new and striking developments in the field of PPD. Probably the most remarkable of these was a report by Ione Railton, M.D., Associate Clinical Professor of Medicine at the University of California School of Medicine in San Francisco.[14] Dr. Railton reported on observations and studies that began in the late 1950s and that were reported in a medical journal in 1961. The reports suggested that a curious aberration of the adrenal glands may be related to severe early PPD (puerperal psychosis), and that this condition may be amenable to rational hormonal treatment. As with many other important findings in the field of PPD, Railton's have gone unnoticed by psychiatrists, and were never verified or disproved by others.

Doctor Railton completed her senior residency in internal medicine in the mid-1950s. She became interested in possible relationships between psychiatric symptoms and medical illnesses, and was granted a fellowship to study these matters at Langley Porter Clinic, the psychiatric service of the University Hospital in San Francisco. At Langley Porter, her attention was attracted by several patients with early, agitated postpartum illness.

As Railton observed, these patients showed marked restlessness, severe insomnia, peculiar trancelike appearance, rapid changes from manic to normal behavior, depression with great anxiety, and fleeting hallucinations and delusions. She was struck by a similarity to a number of patients she had seen on the medical wards, who had been overmedicated with cortisone and then rapidly withdrawn.

In the late 1940s, cortisone, a hormone of the adrenal cortex, was found to be very effective in treating a number of diseases, including painful and disabling conditions such as rheumatoid arthritis. The relief of symptoms was almost magical, and the drug was widely used. Then it was discovered that cortisone could have serious side effects, such as stomach ulcers, diabetes, hypertension, and sometimes undesirable psychiatric symptoms.

When the side effects appeared, cortisone was discontinued. A considerable number of patients developed restlessness, severe insomnia, vague trancelike behavior, manic episodes, depression, and transitory episodes of apparent normality.

In the Department of Medicine at UCSF it had been found that the cortisone-deprived patients could be helped by small doses of prednisolone, a substance related to cortisone. Railton consulted with a distinguished endocrinologist on the staff at UC, Dr. Peter Forsham, secured his guidance and encouragement, and persuaded the chief of the psychiatric service to let her try small doses of prednisolone on early, agitated postpartum patients. The results were very gratifying, and she published a paper in 1961 on sixteen postpartum cases, comparing them with sixteen controls treated only with tranquilizers and sedatives.

Conservative physicians are aware of the fact that no single study constitutes full proof. However, the usual response to an important discovery is that it is tested by others, and gradually established or disproved.

Some physicians at the conference reacted to her report with amazement. Others recognized that if prednisolone was indeed effective, a rational explanation was ready: during pregnancy, total adrenal corticoids are high, up to three times the normal range. However, most of the corticoids are physiologically inactive, bound by an enormous protein molecule. The active free cortisol, possibly representing current production, is a "floater" that comprises roughly 10 percent of the total corticoids. This current production could be low, in response to the sluggish postpartum pituitary. The normal sensor of low cortisol is located in the hypothalamus. If cortisol is very low, and the pituitary adrenals unresponsive to signals from the hypothalamus, the hypothalamus might "explode" and generate many of the symptoms observed in postpartum depression.

A very careful psychiatrist, under the watchful eye of an endocrinologist, might produce remarkable and favorable results with prednisolone. But psychiatrists unskilled in the use of the adrenal steroids and unaware of their hazards could easily administer too-high doses of prednisolone or administer the drug over too long a time and suppress the patient's adrenal glands. There is great concern lest Railton's finding, possibly a major medical discovery, be abused by overeager psychiatrists. Railton's observations must be tested by other researchers. Efforts are being made to encourage this, with her enthusiastic support.

THE PHENOMENON OF HYPOTHALAMIC-PITUITARY COLLAPSE

There is an intriguing postchildbirth drama called *hypothalamic-pituitary collapse,* with short-term and long-term implications. Let us say that the order has gone out from the hypothalamus to the pituitary for more cortisol. The pituitary, having been very active, productive, and with an increased blood supply in pregnancy, has suddenly fallen into a state of relative inactivity, its secretory cells in a resting phase and its circulation greatly diminished since birth. The postpartum pituitary is sluggish. It fails to produce ACTH, which, in turn, would activate the adrenal cortex, thereby generating more cortisol. The level of free *active* cortisol gets lower and lower, the sensor in the hypothalamus responds again, to no avail.

But further external stimuli are hitting the hypothalamus (the center of the body's autonomic nervous system): for example, the mother may be reacting with extreme joy to her newborn, with extreme stress to the nursing and hospital staff, with anger because her husband is late to visit her, with concern for her other children back home—any number of stresses and stimuli that blast the hypothalamus, forcing it to continue its call for cortisol, still with no effect. The victim of this hormonal imbalance begins to have symptoms of emergency reactions: insomnia, fear, palpitations, panic attacks (similar to those brought on by a rush of adrenaline).

Then a catastrophic neurophysiological event occurs: the hypothalamus overreacts, with nerve impulses spreading to areas at some distance from the cortisol sensor, affecting sleep, and the autonomic nervous system. Strange sensations and uncomfortable psychological experiences are activated.

PREVENTION OF PPD

Currently, there are two methods of PPD prevention. One is Katharina Dalton's administration of progesterone, beginning with an injection immediately after delivery and for several days thereafter, followed by progesterone pills for several weeks. She has reported a recurrence rate of 9 percent among seventy-seven women who received progesterone prophylaxis after moderate to severe PPD, against an expected rate of 68 percent among control cases. The results suggest that the administration of progesterone may cushion the normal precipitous fall in progesterone level, thereby forestalling events that could lead to a recurrence.

"I know that progesterone works and that it is safe," Dr. Dalton has said. "Given my way, I would let any woman take it in low doses throughout her reproductive life—I mean for thirty-five years, from the ages of fifteen to fifty—and that way she would never have PMS or PPD. The progesterone we give is natural and has been synthesized from yams. It is not the same as the artificial formula of progestogen used in the Pill [which only helps to reduce levels of the natural progesterone, hence bringing on depression in many women who take the Pill]. No association has been made between this natural hormone and cancer or any other medical problem."

If PPD symptoms develop in the week or two following birth, progesterone cannot be used because the body by then has gone into what Dalton calls the refractory stage (pituitary collapse), and progesterone alone will not trigger the system back into action.

Dalton is a very able and impressive physician. However, some believe that her results might be hard to duplicate with rigid experimental controls. Dalton is the first to suggest that her preventive program should be checked by others.

Another natural substance that may alleviate PPD is the vitamin *pyridoxine,* or B_6, which of course can be purchased from health food stores. The medical and psychiatric professions are following studies of it with keen interest. Dr. Diana Riley, a psychiatrist from Aylesbury, Buckinghamshire, England, presented documented evidence at the 1982 and 1984 Marcé Society conferences. Her most recent study was with a group of fifty-one women who were likely to have a recurrence of PPD and a similar group of controls. They were administered 100 mg of pyridoxine daily for twenty-eight days after delivery. The controls were given a placebo for the twenty-eight-day trial.

Riley's results were convincing enough to make even traditional eyebrows raise. The symptoms of depression in the control group were considerably higher than in the group thought likely to suffer PPD.

Dr. Elisabeth Herz believes there is good reason to think B_6 might be helpful because the vitamin is essential for the synthesis of the neurotransmitters. Riley put forward the notion that the vitamin works directly to correct a deficiency in serotonin uptake (one of the neurotransmitters). Pyridoxine is already in use in Britain and the United States for PMS treatment. As long as the dose does not reach toxic levels—no higher than 200 mg daily, suggested Dr. Herz—the substance is harmless and is likely to be beneficial.

So far, neither of these lines of research has reached standards required of experimental excellence, by which they might be taken on by the remainder of the medical and psychiatric professions. The debate continues over the advisability of running experiments on severely depressed postpartum patients or on those whose conditions might be considered life-threatening. In the meantime, we wait for more funding, more research, and greater interest in the findings. I hope the wait won't take us into the twenty-first century.

ANTIDEPRESSANT MEDICATION

The one area of treatment for PPD that *must* be looked at most carefully, the method of choice for most doctors today (for moderate cases), is *antidepressant medication*. Many women I have spoken with had successfully taken a course of the medication; others had felt no better taking the pills and had given them up; still others had refused even to try them, either not wishing to take a drug in this sensitive period after birth, particularly if they were breast-feeding, or from a deep objection to the possibility that they would become dependent on the pills.

Antidepressants are not to be confused with tranquilizers.[15] They are a successful method of treatment for depression and specifically for PPD. Tranquilizers are *not* a good method of treatment for PPD because they increase fatigue and confused thoughts. Tranquilizers sedate and dull anxiety attacks, but they mask the other symptoms of PPD rather than curing them. Antidepressants, however, are used specifically to *reverse* abnormal brain chemistry, to speed up the flow of those neurotransmitters.

Tranquilizers are sometimes given to women with PPD, but, as with all medications, they should be used sparingly and with caution. In severe cases of postpartum psychosis, when the patient may be very agitated or a danger to herself, a small dose (such as 25 mg) of Thorazine, three times daily, can take the edge off the violence and severe anxiety. Mild doses of a moderate tranquilizer such as Valium can also be a help. But all tranquilizers or sedatives are long-acting and tend to cover up the valuable lucid intervals, during which reassurance to the patient can be most effective. Such use of medication has to be a compromise: the physician must not let the patient destroy herself, yet the medication must be played down so that the new mother does not become a twenty-four-hour zombie, inaccessible to psychotherapy.

Antidepressants are popular among psychiatrists because they work on the brain chemistry but, unfortunately, there is no way of knowing if they are working on the right brain chemistry. So, again, the physician must be encouraged to use as little of the medication as possible at one time, adding to the dosage only if necessary. In a good psychiatric facility, a safe environment and healthy staff attitude can replace a lot of pills. The physician who knows his or her staff can leave "as needed" orders and trust their good judgment. At home, more is demanded of the family and the doctor's personal influence to gain the same objective.

Dr. Herz explained that, in one sense, antidepressants actually resemble vitamin supplements; they, too, make up for a deficiency in our natural systems. In this case, however, the deficiency is in the neurotransmitters themselves. There are three major groups of antidepressants: those commonly known as the tricyclic or tetracyclics (they have three of four chemical rings); the MAOIs (monoamine oxidase inhibitors); and lithium carbonate. The tricyclics are most often used in the United States for PPD, while MAOIs are more common in Europe. Lithium is generally used for recurring depression or mania.

MAOIs appear, logically, to be the perfect course of treatment for PPD, as they work specifically to block an enzyme that renders norepinephrine and serotonin inactive. Dr. Herz explained that MAOIs are used with caution in the United States because doctors fear that the patient may not adhere to strict dietary rules; even minor deviations could lead to hypertensive crisis and ultimately death. The dietary rules are to prevent elevated blood pressure as a reaction to foods containing tyramine: cheese, pickled herring, sausage or other cured meats, and red wine or sherry. MAOIs work quickly, however, taking only ten days to two weeks to reach their full effect.

Prof. George Winokur, of the department of psychiatry at University of Iowa, on the founding committee of the Marcé Society and author of one of the best books on depression for the general public, *Depression: The Facts,* explains that the tricyclics work by blocking the re-uptake of the neurotransmitters serotonin and norepinephrine at the synapses, thereby allowing a greater amount of the neurohormones, so vital to our moods, to be in those all-important spaces between the nerve cells. Some formulas have a more sedating action than others, and doctors will very likely have to experiment with different doses and different brands.[16]

Tricyclic antidepressants may lead to a confused state of mind, dizziness, constipation, fogginess, or skin rash. They take up to three weeks to reach their full effect, and they will reverse the biological abnormality. Ideally, a patient should stay on treatment for several months to prevent a relapse.

Lithium, a naturally occurring substance in the same chemical group as sodium and potassium (one of the salts), has been used successfully for mania for over thirty years. It sedates the hyperactive and may lead to lethargy, but it is not usually prescribed for PPD.

FUTURE TRENDS

So often, serious PPD symptoms have been treated as classical mental illness, from the initial diagnosis right through treatment, and new mothers and their husbands have been left wondering whether these symptoms mean the rest of their lives are going to be affected by PPD; whether any fantasy they may have shared of happy family life will have been crushed. The one main area of change, therefore, that psychiatrists, obstetricians, and scientists would like to see right now is in the treatment of postpartum mothers once they reach the psychiatric wards.

As we have seen with stories like those of Nancy and Barbara, severe symptoms usually get emergency action. The mother is rushed to a psychiatrist or to the hospital, where she will immediately be admitted for treatment and tests; leaving the new father to struggle and cope with the baby, at home.

In Britain, the situation has been different for the past ten years or so. In many major towns and cities there are mother and baby units attached to psychiatric hospitals for admission of the infant with the PPD mother. The first such wing to be tested in the United States is at the Massachusetts Mental Health Center, and more will surely follow in the next few years.[17]

One of Dr. Hamilton's main criticisms of the psychiatric profession and its current handling of PPD is the appalling circumstances that surround the new mother's admission to the hospital. "The ritual admission interrogation, often conducted by an eager staff assistant, involves questions about sexual aberrations and feelings of personal inadequacy. This provides fuel for the fires of hallucination and delusion, and advances the fear of mental breakdown and failure."

Traditionally, mothers were not allowed to bring their infants into the hospital with them because of the archaic assumptions about PPD: (1) the mother's psychiatric problems might lead to an inability to deal with her own hostility toward the child—recovery depended on their separation; (2) the mother was a potential physical and psychological danger to the child; (3) the disturbed behavior of other patients would be harmful to the child; and (4) the presence of young children would be disruptive to the other patients' therapy.[18]

In 1948, Dr. T. F. Main, in Surrey, England, first admitted a mother suffering from PPD into a hospital with her infant. At the time, some hospitals were allowing mothers to stay with infants or young children, because current opinion was concerned with the effects on a *child* of early separation from its mother. But what about the effects on the *mother* of separation from the infant? When that became a focus of interest in the last ten years, units were set up and many interesting studies have emerged.[19]

Ideally, a mother and baby unit would be attached to a psychiatric hospital or in a separate building: it should be a pleasant place, with nursery, playroom, and provision for toddlers as well as infants. There would be outpatient hospital provision, with day care, for those better served by treatment during the day and going home at night. It has been recognized that separation of a mother from her infant, because of PPD, leads to a "gradual slackening in the longing and concern for her child, and precipitates guilt feelings which make resuming motherhood harder."[20]

Better treatment for the most severe cases of PPD (known as postpartum psychosis) has perhaps understandably received the most concentrated effort. Yet even women with these severe cases will still be sent home in a muddle of confused emotions and thoughts if they are not helped to a fuller understanding of their situation.

As the stories in the next chapter illustrate, too many women have received peremptory treatment, often unsympathetic care, and have emerged from their experience of PPD somewhat battle-scarred. It may seem incredible that, in today's sophisticated world, women have been receiving such short shrift from the medical and psychiatric professions, when their problems follow childbirth. These stories must be heard, for the situation has not much improved. As the members of the Marcé Society are quick to emphasize, the scientific community is only at the very beginning of necessary, vital research, and all of its work is still hampered by a general reluctance to accept PPD as a real problem, affecting real women and their families, with a real and urgent need to be studied and more widely understood.

For all the Marcé Society's recent conferences, mailings, support for one another, and occasional encouragement in the form of government grants for new research, they are self-described as a handful of determined men and women trying to keep in touch with one another across the world, when the walls between their separate professions make such communication an enormous obstacle.

Chapter 4

"AM I REALLY CRAZY?"

Severe symptoms of PPD are a pattern of not being able to eat or sleep; high anxiety level or panic attacks; a feeling of being utterly unable to cope; a sluggish depression so deep you cannot get yourself out of bed let alone look after the baby; not being able to bear to touch the baby; constant crying that in itself is disruptive to family life; fear about harming the baby; talk of taking your own life; and a feeling that you are worthless and all would be better off if you were dead.

The severity of such symptoms has led women to describe the effect in words like these: "I thought I was losing my mind," "I cried constantly, screamed at my husband, barely ate or slept, and wanted to die," "I was ashamed, embarrassed, and disgusted with myself. I thought I was going crazy and no one cared," "I felt like I was hanging onto my sanity with my fingernails."

One twenty-eight-year old mother with a one-month-old baby experienced an extreme case of the "distorted crazy" feelings. Helen E. admitted that events had piled up at home, leading to some form of emotional crisis. She had given up work to have the baby, and she missed her job and its financial security. Her husband had used up all their savings to open a new business. There were demands from him to help out, conflicting demands from the baby to be home and be a "real mother," and other demands from family and friends. Helen felt as though she was desperately struggling to keep up a front for everyone. Eventually she could neither eat nor sleep, and she became paranoid.

"One very hot night, I dreamed about the devil. I really believed a demon was trying to get my child," Helen said. Sweating, she had awoken feeling constrained, as though she had a heavy weight on her chest, and there was a buzzing in her head. Helen immediately phoned the family doctor and was referred to the mental health clinic. The psychiatrist there was a rare gem who gave Helen good, reassuring advice. "You are not crazy. You are suffering from PPD." He put her in touch with other women with similar symptoms, offered some therapeutic group sessions, and advised her to avoid all caffeine.

Three stories emerged from my research that, to me, were the most frustrating indications of the inadequacy of treatment and type of attitude that so often prevails with new mothers. Linda S. was viewed as a potential child abuser, and her unsympathetic treatment followed the classic lines of the psychological approach. Adele M. realized long after the event that her depression may not have been totally avoidable, given her personal ambivalence toward having a baby at that time of her life, but still her treatment made it much worse. And Jane L. received what was considered proper treatment, but was left confused and unsure of what had happened, so that, even fifteen years later, she suffers from chronic guilt about her PPD.

Linda: Hormone Imbalance, Not Suicidal Neurosis

Linda's doctors diagnosed her condition, after the birth of her second baby, on strictly psychological grounds. In the words of Gregory Zilboorg, one of the founding fathers of psychiatry, in a paper published in 1957 that is often still quoted, what we supposedly see in women such as Linda is "frigidity and potential homosexuality. . . . We deal here with a castration complex of the revenge type . . . with an unresolved Oedipus situation . . . or with father identification."[21]

Linda and her husband, Tommy, were young and inexperienced parents of two babies eleven months apart. The second child was born shortly before Tommy's departure on a Navy cruise, and Linda knew he would be away for several months; she also knew she just would not be able to cope alone. They had been using contraception and she had not wanted a second baby so quickly. But an IUD failure led to the second baby's conception, delivery was by c-section, and Linda named the infant girl Stephanie, which she remembers thinking was the prettiest name in the world. On recovering from the operation she was overcome by a terrible sadness.

Back home, as the days wore on Linda didn't want to touch Stephanie, or be near her. She could barely manage to feed and clothe her. Linda went to see the Navy chaplain, who reported to Tommy that his wife was unbalanced. Things grew worse, and Linda wanted to put the baby up for adoption. The Navy mental health clinic said they could do nothing to help unless Linda had actually abused her baby. But she wanted help *before* she hurt her. Although they signed adoption papers at one point, the couple panicked and Stephanie was eventually put into foster care along with her year-old brother, Sam.

Linda continued to be treated by the mental health clinic—sometimes with as many as ten pills a day, uppers for daytime and downers to sleep. Her psychiatrist first decided she had lesbian tendencies and then that she hated her mother and father. Even her gynecologist dismissed her feelings that the depression might be due to hormonal imbalance after the birth. But Linda was lucid enough to argue, why would she suddenly start to hate her mother and father now, with the second child? "Why could nobody understand me?" she cried out. The diagnosis on her finally read "neurotic with suicidal tendencies," and she spent fourteen months in and out of that clinic.

About a year later Linda and Tommy were allowed to visit Stephanie in the foster home and sometimes have her to their house as long as Tommy was there to supervise. By then Linda had begun to feel like herself again, and at ease as a mother. "Not from the pills, not from the therapy, but because my body was changing, a feeling of strength was returning," she says. "Yet everyone just assumed I had lost my mind."

Eventually the parents retrieved their children and tried to set up family life again, after a year and a half of torment. Linda reports she has weathered other storms since. She and Tommy were divorced five years later, when she was thirty years old and she had a partial hysterectomy in 1982; she bounced back from both those traumatic events without depression. Linda lost a year of her life and a lot of happiness through poor treatment of PPD. "I sometimes wonder how much simpler it would all have been if I had not just been shrugged off as some neurotic attention-seeking broad."

Linda's overload factor was strong and emphatic: closely spaced children, a husband absent for long periods through his work, few family resources, her age, a youthful, ill-thought-out marriage, a terrifying sense of inadequacy leading to inertia. Her diagnosis as a neurotic with suicidal tendencies failed to make any connection with the psychoendocrine upheaval of birth.

Adele: A Mistaken Psychiatric Diagnosis

Adele M. was a very young, newly married woman, still in college, when she accidentally became pregnant. Horror-struck at first at the thought that she would have to give up college and interrupt her career plans, when she talked it over with Stephen they both came around to the idea of having the baby. They became active in the midwife movement and attended the preparation classes with enthusiasm. Adele and Stephen were both, therefore, disappointed in her emergency c-section delivery but they greeted baby Teddy with joy. All too soon, twenty-three-year-old Adele found her elation disappearing. Nothing had prepared her for the reality of motherhood: she was now out of school and living miles away from parents or friends, surrounded by what she felt were hostile neighbors, and coping with Teddy, who was a difficult baby. She said, "Boredom and loneliness soon set in with the guilt and feelings of inadequacy."

Adele saw a family doctor, who reassured her that the problem was hormonal, the baby blues, and that things would soon get better. But within a week Adele was hardly functioning. Desperate, Stephen took her to a psychiatrist. Adele was drugged senseless and admitted immediately to a hospital. On reflection, Adele has realized that her depression might not have been totally avoidable, given her degree of ambivalence toward motherhood in the first place, but it need not have been so severe or as badly handled. She was hospitalized for nine months, a long time for PPD, leaving Stephen and her mother, who had to come live in their house, to deal with Teddy.

The hospital psychiatrist asked her over and over again about her childhood and any sexual problems. "Finally my mother convinced Stephen that this was not brought on by some childhood trauma, that nothing had happened to me sexually, and that maybe we should try a different doctor because she felt I should be home with Teddy. We saw a new doctor and, you know, his attitude was so different. He just said, 'How soon did the problem come on after the birth?' Then he took me off all medications and sent me home with a list of phone numbers of women in similar circumstances in the area. Part of my problem had been the isolation. I had had no car and felt cut off from anyone like myself."

Stephen understood more about his wife's condition, and they decided together to borrow the money to buy a car so that Adele could return to college, meet with these other mothers, and not suffer the trapped, isolated feelings of new motherhood. It was a family approach to psychotherapy. Care, concern, and an understanding doctor achieved what nine months of heavy psychoanalysis and medication had not even touched.

A year later, Adele had adjusted but was aware enough to recognize that motherhood could still be hard for her; that mealtimes, bedtimes, and potty training were stresses she did not find easy. But at least she could now admit to this supposed failure. "Being a good mother and wife, I learned, meant taking care of *me*, too."

She had joined the cesarean-section prevention movement, was busy with her school work, enjoyed an aerobics class, and was happier with Teddy. Adele felt she could even imagine having another baby, knowing that if things grew bad again she had somewhere to turn for support. Adele's final plea was, why can't there be local PPD groups for new mothers to belong to? Why not indeed?

Jane: A Case of Fatigue and Hopelessness

Jane L.'s symptoms of PPD came after the birth of her second baby. She was a working sculptor who had continued to be productive through her first child's early years. Her husband, Jim, was a specialist in an international field and could be called away from home at one week's notice for three-month intervals. What is interesting is that neither Jane nor the considerate Jim had thought to look into the implications of his being away when she had young children to look after.

With the first child, Kim, Jane had gone to Hong Kong to join Jim, and they had lived there for nearly a year. Jane kept up with her work. When they returned to the States, a much-wanted second pregnancy had begun. It was an easy pregnancy and even easier birth, which, to their delight, they were able to have at home. But the new baby, Jesse, was not the dream baby his sister, Kim, had been. Jesse was born crying and screaming, and although Jane determined to breast-feed him, he never seemed satisfied. "Maybe it was the three-and-a-half year gap, but I just didn't feel I could cope with it all, this time. I was soon overwrought and overfatigued, and I slumped into a typical type of PPD lethargy, dullness, and mild despair."

Jane was given antidepressants by a family doctor, but then Jim was called away to work in the Caribbean. They arranged that she would fly out with the children, in a couple of months' time, to join him for Christmas. This left Jane with the two young children in a rented house (an "idyllic country cottage"—remote, isolated, and lonely) where supposedly she would paint and revel in the joys of motherhood, miles away from family or any friends.

Endeavoring to pack for their departure, dealing with the isolation, fatigue, and despair, less able to cope because the antidepressants were making her drowsy and confused, Jane decided in late October to put the kids in the car and drive a hundred miles to visit her family. Her mother was ill and she wanted to see her; she also had a married sister and brother in the vicinity. (Jane's father had been a manic depressive all his life, but Jane and her siblings had been continually advised it was not hereditary. Indeed, only now can Jane see that maybe she shared some personality traits with this man she had scarcely known.)

It was not easy staying with relatives with six-month-old Jesse, who was teething, and screaming loudly. The visit turned into a major stressor, as Jane argued with her sister and then felt fear for her mother. The fatigue and feeling of not being able to cope grew worse and worse. She was getting little sleep and was very overwrought. So Jane put the kids back in the car and began the drive home to their rented house.

It was pouring rain and the car broke down on the highway, but she handled that emergency even though Jesse was screaming in his car seat behind her. Wracked with exhaustion, Jane just said to herself, "Plough on, we'll be there soon." But she began to find it harder to peer through the gloom, half-blinded by the other car headlights. Suddenly she knew she could not go on. Jane pulled into a service station and begged for help. The local police were called in, and they tried to contact her family, but neither brother nor sister could come out to help her just then. The police suggested she check into a motel for the night and get some sleep, and they arranged for her brother to pick her up the next morning.

"Why am I being such a bother? Why can't I look after myself?" she was angrily thinking to herself.

That night in the motel room, trying to get the children to sleep by reading them a story, she knew she was cracking up. "My thoughts and thought processes were in turmoil. The wires were jumbled up. I was in a state of panic. I started to fantasize reading the story and it was becoming real to me."

Her brother drove them back to their mother's home. A family doctor gave Jane a sedative to make her sleep all night. But she woke still confused, delirious, helplessly crying. Jane was admitted to the nearby psychiatric hospital. Jesse was sent to stay with his paternal grandparents (in their seventies) and Kim stayed on with the sick maternal grandmother. In her wildest dreams Jane could not have envisioned a worse situation for her children, or for her family. But everything had been taken out of her hands. The body and the mind had given up, knowing they could not cope.

Jane was in a psychiatric hospital for nearly two months. She does not remember much, apart from the four electric shock (ECT) treatments. Heavily sedated, she could hardly think most of the time. Her mother made perhaps the worst mistake, telephoning Jim in the Caribbean and telling him, "Oh no, don't rush home, everything's fine." Jane remained confused, distorted, deeply guilty, and embarrassed throughout her hospital stay. In January, when Jim returned, she recalls, "He walked into the hospital, was patient, kind, concerned, and very sweet to me. Within ten days I was out of there."

Jane's treatment worked, maybe by default. Properly given, ECT may be very effective and not the disturbing treatment for depression of the old days. But Jane may not have needed even the ECT had her real condition been understood earlier. During her stay in a psychiatric hospital, she had received no psychotherapy. No one ever sat down with her and talked about motherhood, about her responsibilities; about how she felt coping alone with her husband away, how she felt about being a mother. As Jane put it, "I never sorted out what it might be. It was such a dramatic thing to happen yet I never understood it. My husband and I never talked about it. It just came and went, like in a vacuum. It has taken me years to get over the guilt."

Jane's story should at least remind fathers of young children that they *must* play a strong, supportive, and near-equal role in the care of their family. It is really cruel to expect a wife to be able to cope just because that's what women have always done. The truth has only recently been emerging: that most women *cannot* cope alone, especially if they are isolated from family and friends, with little money, other resources, or outside activities.

Jane's was a classic case of lack of sleep, of feeling unable to cope, overwrought, inadequate as a mother, and helplessly alone. The overload factors for her would be obvious to an enlightened observer. Because those around her could not, or would not, see it, her biochemistry finally took over in a complete physical and mental collapse.

Biochemical upheaval does not come from a void: it is not willed on us by a bad fairy. All human bodies, male or female, are carefully balanced frameworks of the body and mind. The hormonal changes of childbirth can and will lead to mental and emotional changes if there are heavy or unexpected stresses on our psyches. In Part Two, I explore more fully just what those pressures might be. We all have within us the vulnerability to crack under great strain. Unfortunately, that vulnerability may not become evident until after the birth.

PART TWO

Why Do I Feel Like This When I Should Be So Happy?

Chapter 5

YOUR CHANGING SENSE OF SELF

We come to parenting from very different backgrounds than any of our female predecessors. It is unlikely we were raised solely to be housewives and mothers; very likely that we held a job for several years. Whether this was the beginning of a career or merely a means of awaiting marriage and motherhood, it gave us independence, our own money, a sense of self, and the use of our own time.

In our childless days we led busy lives: long hours out of the home at work, maybe exercise classes or evening classes, running at dawn or dusk, time to spend with friends and with lovers or new husbands. There was probably travel, and self-indulgent shopping for furniture and clothes. Our marriages were formed with time for each other, with neatly revolving lives as two adults went about their business.

Traditionally, women have sacrificed anything and everything on becoming a mother. But that tradition is weakening. Women are voicing discomfort at the lack of freedom they discover with motherhood, at their inability to fit into the role of mother as even they had perceived it. The psychological stress derived from a poor connection between preconceived notions of how we will be as a mother and the rather different reality will lead to that other cause of PPD: the conflicts of postparenthood adaptation. Like caged animals used to roaming free in the forest, new parents must learn to function and move in more limited space. They must learn to suppress the ego, the desire to do as they please, the self-indulgence, and learn to blend their whole being and psyche with another's. That is not easy.

Child- and baby-care books tend to gloss over this all-too-vital adaptation by the new parents. It is not an adjustment, for that would imply something temporary until the former self could return. Some books indeed offer ideal images of very sane, mature, conscientious parents adjusting to each other's needs, adapting marital, personal, social, and sexual demands to the new stresses and strains of parenting. In reality the two people are probably fighting their way out of a deep pit that threatens to engulf them. The struggle that many go through at this crucial time is for survival of the self, for identity, for a new motivation to carry them through life.

What surprises me is not that we adults find this adaptive process difficult but that, as sensible adults, we expect it to be easy. Do any of us view adolescence or middle age as simple journeys from one life stage to another? Why, I wonder, has it remained an acceptable view that crossing into parenthood is a nontraumatic step? Some recognition of the major risks involved should definitely be part of our new parenthood manifesto, so we can say, with the bumper sticker I saw the other day, "Being a parent is not easy!"

We must bear in mind that the growth stages from single to parent are complex, divisive, potentially destructive, and as deep as any we will have traversed in our own lives since puberty or the early teens.

Unfortunately, I have no magic diets or exercise regimes that will banish overnight the blues or depression; instead, I want to confront the psychological stressors that are an integral part of PPD, working on the neuroendocrinological system. It is the body's overload factor, the final blackout of the system, that will plunge a mother into PPD. But the trigger may well have come from subconscious or conscious stresses loading extra work and energy on the postpartum vulnerable metabolic balance. These demands come at just the wrong time, when the mother does not have the strength or emotional support to meet the new needs.

AMBIVALENCE

Let us look at a very tricky concept, the natural ambivalence everyone feels on becoming a parent. In theory, pregnancy gives mothers at least nine long months of mental time not only to buy baby clothes and furnish the nursery but to work out her relationship and attitude to having a child. But there are so many conflicting emotions and thoughts to work through, I doubt many give it that much conscious thought.

One of the paradoxes of ambivalence is that when a pregnancy is *chosen,* we tend to turn around full circle and in place of arguments against having babies, we can only think of arguments *for.* I know I had been quite antichildren: in the mid- to late 1960s it was from fear of the bomb—who would ever bring up children in such a dangerous world? In the early 1970s, there was zero population growth to work for as an ideal, and people who had babies were seen as selfishly destroying the world. By the mid-1970s, feminism emerged with its own brand of arguments, that women would not have babies until men learned to help them care for them, until men would take time off work for childcare. I had written magazine articles citing reasons why women did not have to have children, and why they should fight the cultural pressures to become mothers.

Then my own biological cravings overcame all that logic. From my late twenties until I finally had my first baby at age thirty-one, I was often reduced to a crying mass of confusion: did I really want to have a baby; could I possibly cope with raising a child; would I ever meet a man I felt would offer the protection and support necessary; if not, would I have a baby on my own? Those questions must afflict many women today. But then I met the man, and he too wanted to start a family. A thunderbolt had struck me, and in so doing managed to block out those anxious, warning, overcautious brain cells; I forgot all my arguments against, and desperately looked forward to having a baby. When ambivalence is so firmly pushed to the back of the mind, it lurks, deceivingly, waiting to creep back up front when there is a gap in the mind's protective devices, to feed disquiet again at a later date. The truth is that ambivalence felt before, even if forgotten during the optimism of pregnancy, is obviously a part of our *whole* self. It can and does return.

Book editor Anne P., having her baby in her late thirties, finally made the decision with her husband that they would try to conceive. Imagining she would have some problem, they expected at least a year of trying to conceive and time to get used to the idea of being parents. She became pregnant the first month. Her instant reaction was total elation, that she had passed the test of fertility and femininity. The elation was followed shortly by panic: "How am I ever going to be a mother when I can't even look after myself?" That was followed by ambivalence: "Of course I want a baby, but I don't want to give up my former life."

We learn to live with the ambivalence, accept it as part of our lives. Some of us with a strong sense of self and humor hide the feelings in a kind of cynical humor. But, if the ambivalence is too heavy, for whatever reason, it can easily lead to a deep-rooted despair that we are not good mothers because we are not living up to our own fantasized image of the sort of mother we should be.

THE FEELING OF ENTRAPMENT

I was moved by the confessional outpourings in the letters I received. Many women expressed openly some of the shock they had experienced on becoming mothers. Sometimes having had a baby made them feel they were trapped, tied down, enslaved again, as though the freedoms of the modern world had vanished overnight, leaving them in that traditional situation of women, mothers, of the past. They were mourning that "free" self of their own pasts; but rather than mourning that past with simple grief, these mothers were confused by a terrible guilt that good mothers would never, ever, feel such emotions.

Admitting to feeling trapped by motherhood seems to take a lot of courage and strength in the face of social judgments that mothers should not complain. Indeed, other mothers may frown to hear such comments; pediatricians or obstetricians might suggest, subtly or overtly, that the mother has no right to such feelings. The new mother who might be suffering mild early warning signs of PPD will withdraw into her protective shell, stay silent, and believe the problems are hers alone, caused only by her inadequacy. Entrapment, however, is a normal, obvious, common experience after childbirth. It's a physical sensation as well as mental or emotional. After the birth of my second child, I felt as though I had literally grown another limb; a limb that was deadweight and had to be dragged around behind me every waking minute. I could not run to the store, go to an exercise class, or choose to meet a friend without arranging, planning, negotiating my time. I cannot imagine the new mother who would not be affected by the strictures on her self and her freedom.

As Nancy E. put it, "Motherhood does take away a lot of your freedom. It is a lot of work, and a lot of responsibility, and if any woman says that isn't frightening and a sobering thought, I don't think she is being honest."

When Nancy E. first wrote to me, she had to enclose a covering note. She had poured her heart out to me in seven typewritten pages and now she said that doing so had made her break down again. Just to read what she had written reminded her of the pain. Several days had now passed, and she had been able to read it without falling apart. This, she felt, was progress!

Nancy had grown up in a large family, in a rural setting, always knowing she wanted to be a housewife and mother. With her first daughter she had gone back to teaching, but had gladly given that up when her husband began his own business and she could work a couple of days a week for him. Finally, she was able to fulfill her idealized picture of herself—a real mother, baking cookies and all the rest of it.

It was obviously a shock to have to admit she felt trapped by her new life once her second baby was born. Recently she had gone back to helping in her husband's business two days a week, which got her out of the house and back to a semblance of herself again.

"It has helped alleviate the feeling of being trapped and the panic attacks which followed. I still have bad days when I'm overcome with a sensation of panic, and then guilt. I have to remind myself that I still do have a life of my own, that it really won't be that long before the baby is old enough to be truly portable."

Few experts have really understood that mothers genuinely suffer this trapped feeling. In one of Dr. Benjamin Spock's books, *Problems of Parents,* in a section called "Mothers Need a Break Too," Spock endeavored to explain why mothers complain to their doctors about feeling confined and lonely.[22]

In this book, which was originally published in 1962, his view was that women who worked before marriage did so without a sense of commitment and always with an escape hatch. If they were bored at work, they would leave one day when the right man came along. Therefore, unlike men, they had an "illusory sense of freedom." When they had their first baby, the escape hatch seemed to bang shut, and he obviously felt their complaints were the reaction of someone who was spoiled. He pointed out that no one had forced these women into marriage and childbearing; most of them had spent their youthful years dreaming and wanting such a future.

In the most up-to-date Spock (with Dr. Michael Rothenberg), *Baby and Child Care,* which new mothers still turn to for reassurance and guidance, Spock's section called "Parents" has subtitles such as "Parents Are Human" and "Parental Doubts Are Normal." In "Mixed Feelings About Pregnancy," he certainly updates that archaic notion about women and their right to a sense of freedom. "We have an ideal about motherhood that says that a woman is overjoyed when she finds that she is going to have a baby. When it arrives she slips into the maternal role with ease and delight. This is all true to a degree—more in one case, less in another. But it is of course only one side of the picture. Medical studies have brought out (what wise women have known all along) that there are normal negative feelings connected with a pregnancy, too, especially the first one.

"To some degree, the first pregnancy spells the end of carefree youth—very important to Americans. The maidenly figure goes gradually into eclipse, and with it goes sprightly grace. . . . The woman realizes that after the baby comes there will be distinct limitations of social life and other outside pleasures. No more hopping into the car on the spur of the moment, going anywhere the heart desires, and coming home at any old hour. . . ."[23]

There are two pages in *Baby and Child Care* on feeling blue. Spock believes that it is common for mothers to feel discouraged, weep easily, and feel bad about certain things after the birth. "There are all the physical and glandular changes at the time of birth, which probably upset the spirits to some degree." Then he adds, "The majority of mothers don't get discouraged enough in this period even to call it depression."[24] Dr. Spock, I must send you some of the letters I received!

Dr. Guttmacher, in devoting one paragraph to the blues in *Pregnancy, Birth and Family Planning,* maintains that periods of crying and depression are common to new mothers and he advises a woman to discuss it frankly with her doctor, who can "reassure you that he has met postpartum blues many times in stable, well-adjusted, fundamentally happy people, whose depression cleared up in a few days without aftermath or treatment."[25]

More contemporary pregnancy books have devoted some space to women's emotional and psychological adjustment after birth.[26] Many, however, offer advice that really lacks depth of information. The most they offer is the belief that positive thinking will banish the blues or we can work our way out of that mythical "learned helplessness."

It was that type of comment, available in pregnancy and child-care books, that had so offended many of my correspondents who, once PPD really hit them, were anxiously seeking guidance or reassurance in the books that had helped them with all the other problems of pregnancy and the first few months of baby care.

LOSS OF IDENTITY

There is a strange sinking feeling that your ego has been submerged in the baby's, that you have been completely taken over and possessed. Pediatric authors Klaus and Kennell, in their book *Maternal-Infant Bonding*, coined the term "enlargement" to describe the baby's image in our minds becoming huge, grand, larger than life, as though he or she were a giant and we were a mere speck.[27] The authors feel it is possibly a necessary part of bonding. I wonder if it might also be a subconscious expression of the fear that our ego has been swamped.

Many women complain after a birth that their bodies have changed, seemingly irrevocably. At the simplest level, their misery may be over weight gain and an inability to fit into clothes from a former lifestyle. Gaining too many extra pounds does lead to a very real problem in losing that weight. It leads, too, to a confused self-image, and fear they are no longer sexual beings. It can mean they literally lose sight of themselves.

Dianne McL. weighed 220 pounds when she gave birth to her daughter at age thirty. Part of her crying in the hospital was the embarrassment at being unable to look after her baby properly and at her body size. "When you're pregnant," she said, "you are magical and holy. Then all of a sudden you're a big lump of pain and anxiety, and you have a baby with a mouth open to satisfy. You have no identity. You don't look or feel what you were before."

Another young, very active woman Gaynor T. described feeling no longer herself: "My firm breasts were replaced with sagging flabby ones which were much smaller. My thin waist and flat tummy were bigger and flabby. My narrow hips were wider," said Gaynor. At twenty-four, a teacher, she had always been busy with dancing, aerobics, working out at the gym, and jogging. "Yet these disturbing changes to my body didn't go away no matter how hard I worked out."

Many women experience a period after birth when they don't know what to wear any more. Their sense of clothes, of personal style, seems to have vanished. They really don't know who they are and what clothes would reflect that image. Many new mothers complain they live in jeans and T-shirts. *After all, babies are messy and who am I dressing for anyway?* Are these silly, vain, purely female, responses? I don't believe so. All women experience them to some degree. It is the reality behind the psychological jargon. It takes time, not to adjust but to transmute: to emerge from the chrysalis into a new person.

Another sense of loss we go through is for the child in us, the little girl we once were; the little girl we suddenly know can never come back. It is not easy to grow up, incontrovertibly, overnight. Something must be left inside of us crying, "But who will look after me?" We are saddened because of the loss; we feel scared, panic-stricken. When her mother finally went home after staying a few days to help out with the baby, one new mother left all on her own wept just as though it was her first day at kindergarten and her mother had left her.

Dianne McL. wrote of this emotionally vulnerable time in a journal, "I remember before I had the baby, taking a walk with my small dog. It seems when I look back that is when my depression started. I walked up the street leading to my house, a fully ripened piece of fruit, but still one person, independent, carefree at nine months pregnant.

"I remember thinking this may well be the last time I can leave the house alone and enjoy a walk on a summer's evening without a care, with no one else to consider. I remember trying to savor the moment. It brings tears to my eyes now to think of that moment, of that freedom. Somehow your carefree days of youth are over, once you have a child."

Losing the little girl can also make us feel much older. Kathy S. was twenty-six when she had baby Joe. Although she knew she was not old, becoming a mother suddenly represented feeling like her own mother. "She was thirty-three when she had me, so it was not even as though we were the same age." But for Kathy, being like her mother meant being tied down with responsibilities, being unhappy, being middle-aged.

Nancy E. also felt that having her second baby at thirty-one forced her to feel old. At twenty-five, with her first baby, she said, "I knew I'd still be young when she grew up a bit. But with Val I felt I'd never be young again. I felt life passing me by. It seems like more of a sacrifice once you're in your thirties. By the time Val is in school I'll be nearly forty. When you're younger, you're content to sit around with other mothers over coffee. But I don't want to waste my life like that any more."

MYTHS OF MOTHERHOOD

The biggest myth we have let ourselves believe, the hardest fairy tale to banish from our collective mythology, is that motherhood comes to every woman by instinct and that our very chromosomes programmed us to be good mothers. This naturally nurturing self-image we project is our most vulnerable point after childbirth.

The fantasized self-image of how we will look, be, and act as a mother has dangerous consequences. A girl grows up believing that one day she will be a mother. If she does become one, every aspect of her self-worth, gender identification, and sense of identity, whether she is chairman of the board at IBM or an avid homemaker can be crushed in seconds if she feels she does not fit that fantasized image. Her fear then leads to the complex assumption she is not a good mother and therefore that she is a failure as a woman.

Dr. Herz emphasized, "Mothering is a learning process, which we have to repeat with each child. The saddest part is that in our attempt to overcome what may be a wrong notion, we usually end up thinking there is something wrong with *ourselves.*" Self-confidence, she pointed out, crashes quickly and easily under stress, and it is hard to rebuild. A diminished self-image contributes to many a case of PPD.

It is certainly incredible that very few hospitals offer women actual courses in basic baby care and handling. The lecture given to the crowd of new mothers, when I had my first baby, on how to bathe your newborn was performed on a plastic doll (whose head did not act as though it would fall off). Diapering cannot be learned from a diagram. Breast-feeding can easily become a nightmare if the mother is tense and feels inadequate, with nurses pushing and pulling and the baby screaming. And who teaches us how to get proper sleep with a baby who cries all the time?

That sense of inadequacy as a mother is perhaps the most

common trigger for PPD. For example, Laura S. had suffered a bad attack of "not being a good or a real mother." She says, "I had read up all about infertility, imagining it would take me up to six months to get pregnant, because I was so much the tense working woman. But I got pregnant the first time. I realize now I didn't know the *first thing* about babies or mothering.

"But I approached my pregnancy right. I was the model pregnant person, going to exercise classes, to the right maternity dress shops for pregnant-executive clothes. Nick and I attended Lamaze classes. I thought I looked great. I carried no extra weight and worked right up to the day before delivery. I'd read everything I could on pregnancy, labor, and breastfeeding, and was determined I'd do it right. I even arranged with the nurse at work that I'd go downstairs and pump my breasts during the work day.

"I had a great delivery. We had a boy, which both of us wanted. And then I saw this kid. And I didn't know what to do with it. I panicked. I'm not a selfish person. I'm Italian, from a large extended family, but still I have never been the type to hang around other people's babies. My mind was still focused on work and what I had to do before I went back in. (I had planned to attend some business meetings the very next week!) I didn't know what it was but I started crying right there in the hospital and I couldn't stop."

BREAST-FEEDING PROBLEMS

Laura had problems with breast-feeding. Before Bobby was born she had read everything on breast-feeding and was sure that's what she would do. "I never felt the milk come in. There I was, expecting so much of myself and I had no milk. It just created more tension in me. All the other women in the hospital were heavier than me. I was slim. But I had no milk, while they were flowing everywhere. I felt like such a failure.

"It became an obsession with me to make it work. I had equipment at home—breast pumps and all. The doctor said to relax. I tried everything. I gave up after two weeks. He was feeding every hour and a half, always hungry, crying, quite miserable.

"Because I was going back to work early, the depression worsened. I had invested everything in being able to nurse my child. In six weeks, I thought, I'll walk out of here and leave him with a caretaker. I'm not even breast-feeding, so what am I to this baby? I'm not really his mother."

Laura continued to have problems with her self-image well into the first year of Bobby's life. Was she a real mother? She could not nurse the baby. She went out to work all day and left him with a caretaker. She had no desire to stay home with him in place of work. Who and what was she? Just a receptacle who had carried him into life?

Bobby cried a lot when they got him home. He was never a contented baby. Other women were strolling around, fat and flowing with milk, with fat, happy babies. Laura had lost the weight she gained with no problem. She was thin and elegant. But she had no milk, and her baby screamed. "I felt a complete failure as a mother," she said.

Failure with breast-feeding seems to be devastating to many women. Marsha H. described the horror of turning baby Jason's head to her breast, stroking his cheek as she had been taught, only to find him turning away. There had been chaos in the couple of days after her c-section delivery, with more surgery needed, but nothing was as bad as this experience.

"He cried desperately and the more he cried the more uptight I became. The nurses said things like, "You've got to get the better of him," and I felt awful. I was thirty-five years old, I'd been a working woman all my life. It just felt like I was not made to be a mother. My emotions were pulled apart. I'd been so looking forward to it all. I was the laughing stock of the hospital. I'm sure they saw me as a middle-age, bossy woman who was too old to be starting it all.

"The feeding did settle down, but the pressure and anxiety over the battle must have had an impact on my psyche. When you're used to being competent in the working world it's even worse to feel like such a *failure* at something that should be so easy."

It was clear to me that even before pregnancy Marsha saw herself as a working woman, as an older mother, and therefore not as a real mother. I'm not suggesting that those inner feelings caused the feeding problem, but combined they triggered a depression.

I know that feeling well—the "I'm not feminine enough to breast-feed my baby" syndrome. When my first was born, I suffered a similar alienation from myself. After a c-section I was running a temperature, and I was not allowed to hold or nurse my baby for nearly a week. She was bottle-fed in the nursery or by my husband. (My hospital roommate made sure I used the electric pump.)

When I was handed my baby six days later I was terrified of her. Of course she wouldn't want my breast milk, I felt. What had I got to offer her—I wasn't a real mother. But my roommate said gently, "Don't be afraid, she's yours, no one else's. All she wants to do in the world is suckle the breast. There's no competition involved, it's natural to her. She's just a little animal." If one person had looked at me critically, if one nurse had hovered, trying to give instructions, I would have given my daughter a bottle rather than face the humiliation.

We have given ourselves new pressures these days: on top of the fear of failure if we do not give birth naturally, without pain, there is also the fear of not being an earth-mother, flowing with milk. Some of us do find breast-feeding exhausting, limiting, a strain. Our babies cry all the time, we get no sleep, our nerves are frayed, we do not make enough milk, everyone in the house is irritable, and yet we feel we must persevere. To my mind, we should not make breast-feeding into a battle to succeed. If the baby would be happier on the bottle, we would be happier too. If our husbands prefer us to bottle-feed so they can truly share some of the duties, both of us would be happier. We are not in the birthing business to be tested, compete, score points off one another. Babies cannot be given *all* the priorities. They are going to be grown-ups themselves one day.

The Colic Crisis: Nancy

Could any of us ever be mentally or emotionally prepared for the worst forms of colic, or screaming babies? The childcare books try to give advice, that soothing, calming, or keeping the baby stimulated will help. But if colic hits your home for three months or more, devastation will be the name of the game: an exhausted mother and a strained marital relationship bear the brunt of the crisis.

Nancy E.'s story of the crying baby trauma, her desperate attempts to continue breast-feeding, and her ultimate breakdown should be a lesson to us all. The former elementary school teacher had an overload on her emotions even before the birth of Val. Nancy's marriage to her husband meant taking on his four children (at the time of their marriage, a boy of ten, six-year-old twins, and a two year old). Nancy's own first baby, Annie, had been a model child and, after putting her on the bottle, she went quickly back to teaching because they then needed the money.

Eight years later, the second baby was due, with the disapproval of Nancy's mother-in-law, who was extremely critical of this plan to further drain her son's finances. Around the same time the elder boy had begun to be a difficult teenager. But the pregnancy went fine and delivery was easy. When they brought Val home, eight-year-old Annie adored her. Nancy felt she had the whole world by the tail.

Val cried through the first two nights and had to be hospitalized again for jaundice. Nancy was soon exhausted. She caught the flu, became dehydrated, and worried that her milk was drying up. Back home from the hospital, Val continued to cry constantly. The more Nancy tried to nurse her, the more the baby cried.

In the middle of this tense situation, her husband, David, was rushed to hospital for minor surgery. Her stepson flunked out of college and left them a note saying it was all their fault. The mother-in-law felt justified in her criticisms. Nancy began to blame the chaos on herself. Even without the colic and consequent lack of sleep, Nancy's overload factors were probably already causing an undue strain on her precarious metabolic balance after the birth.

Through it all, Val continued screaming. "I knew I didn't have enough milk," said Nancy. "Sometimes she would nurse for one and a half hours and would still be crying with frustration. I tried watching everything I ate, drinking beer, eating brewer's yeast. We even drove hours one night to a hospital so I could sniff oxytocin to help let the milk down. By the time Val was ten weeks old, our home had become unbearable. Every day was pure hell, with the baby screaming, and me trying to nurse, and blaming myself for ruining our happy family.

"I stopped being able to eat. I stopped being able to sleep. One morning, at 6 A.M., after being up all night pumping my breasts, I fell apart. When I begged my husband to help me, he responded, 'For heaven's sake, stop this.' But by then even he could see it was serious. He called the obstetrician, who put me on Seconal, and I slept. They had to bottle-feed Val. Within twenty-four hours she was a different baby. She fed and napped, and slept all night."

What help had Nancy received from advisers on her breast-feeding problem? She felt afterward that she would like to strangle the local La Lèche League, who made her feel guilty enough to continue with the struggle at all costs. Her friends gave her grief, telling her how awful bottle-feeding is. Her pediatrician took it upon himself to pressure her into continuing despite her exhaustion.

"My pediatrician's opinion was I had a tense baby, and I should let her cry. He advised me to hold her, to make eye contact. He actually said if I stopped breast-feeding, I'd have *nothing* to comfort her with, that things would be *worse.* He arranged for a counselor to come visit me and the baby, to help me handle the crying. She would hold the baby until the screaming had stopped, and then say, 'There, that's all she needed. See, the tension has gone.' But I couldn't hold my baby for hours like that, while she screamed. And as soon as the counselor left, the screaming would start up again."

Nancy collapsed from exhaustion, frustration, anxiety, lack of sleep, and emotional devastation. Unfortunately, this was only the beginning of a long, deep depression for her, triggered as we now know by her body's inability to restore enough hormones to deal with the extreme anxiety, tension, and fears of her personal inadequacy in a crisis situation. Was it the baby's colic that was at fault? Or was Nancy's tension partly a cause of the colic? There are so many different arguments and theories about the cause of colic, often offered not only by relatives and friends but by pediatricians too, that a sensitive and vulnerable mother can easily be deeply offended by some of the comments.

Another mother, whose child is now a teenager, recalled that when this baby boy was suffering from colic she read an article in a major magazine saying that extensive research with monkeys had proven that colic resulted from inadequate mothering from a tense, nervous, unconfident mother. A lot of people, including doctors, seem to believe this still: it is hard to shift from our deep subconscious, along with those other myths of motherhood, the idea that a good mother naturally and instinctively knows what is best for her baby. As this woman admits, she was devastated by the article and happily let her aunt, who had come to help her care for the infant, take over. The aunt used old-fashioned wisdom, bottle-fed the baby on a four-hour schedule, and cured him rapidly. She claimed that colicky babies had poor digestion and could not deal with the demand schedules that are popularly believed to be best for babies. The baby did in fact have lots of gas and a belly that was absolutely rigid during an attack. No doubt members of the La Lèche League and similar advocates of total breast-feeding would disagree. Many parents who have bottle-fed their babies have also suffered through colic.

The best advice for mothers undergoing problems, either with breast-feeding or with a colicky baby, is that they must focus on their own anguish, their own loss of self-esteem and fears that they are a failure as a mother, rather than worry about the baby. Lack of sleep, lack of self-confidence, lack of any private time or sense of oneself are all major triggers for PPD, as the body and the brain struggle to cope with the overload of demands placed upon them.

In a very helpful new book, *Crybabies: Coping with Colic, What to Do when Baby Won't Stop Crying,* Dr. Marc Weissbluth, director of the sleep disorders center at the Children's Memorial Hospital in Chicago, tries to explain that parents really should be doing less rather than more to overcome colic or extreme crying in newborns.[28] He now believes, after extensive research, that some babies cry more than others mainly because of a confused sleep pattern. Their crying, therefore, does not mean that they are suffering acute indigestion, reacting to your diet, responding to your inadequacy or tension, or a multitude of other reasons that have been proffered over the centuries. They are really crying because they cannot get to sleep. The parents' best form of help might indeed be to let the baby alone, try not to let the crying bother them, and wait till sleep finally takes over. How strange that after decades of theories and controversy, the newest expert opinion should go back to the oldest wives' tale. I remember my mother telling me how, when I was a baby, I was left down at the end of the garden in a carriage (on fine days, no doubt) to cry it out. Nobody picked babies up, caressed them, or made eye-to-eye contact with them to defeat tension. We survived.

Dr. Weissbluth ends his book with the following advice, under the heading What Should I Do?

"Dear parents, when your baby is crying, do nothing. But do nothing deliberately, quietly, gently, confidently and *firmly.* In other words, please try to develop an attitude of:

Purposeful inattention
Studied inattentiveness
Gentle firmness
Constructive resignation
Expectant observation
Watchful waiting

Be attentive to your baby's behavior at night, but try to cultivate a detached and relaxed attitude. As you have read, it does work!"[29]

Chapter 6

BEFORE AND AFTER LAMAZE

CHILDBIRTH EXPERIENCES

We have become thoroughly involved, in recent years, with the perfection of pregnancy, the birth experience, and motherhood; yet we tend to overlook the crushing effect this drive toward perfection can have on us. Attending childbirth education classes, learning breathing and relaxation techniques, insisting to our doctors that we have a drug-free labor, taking special care with our diets and behavior during pregnancy, taking every precaution for the health and safety of the unborn child, we expect and demand pain-free labor and delivery. I don't quite see how women can stop this urge to perfection in the birth experience. How can we change our attitude so the resulting anticlimax when a c-section is ordered (for good medical reasons) will be accepted as a simple disappointment, without the concurrent hostility and resentment directed at the doctor and anger at ourselves?

Expectations of perfect natural childbirth, and the ensuing disappointment, are major triggers, in many women, of PPD. A sense of personal failure emerges that is so huge and long-lasting, so irrational and emotional, that the resulting depression may last for up to a year. Self-help groups for c-section mothers have proved useful, enabling women to get together and vent their feelings, to discuss and share their mourning for the natural birth experience they so looked forward to and expected of themselves. More emphasis in childbirth preparation classes would also be helpful in explaining just why c-sections may be necessary, what they entail, and why the mother should prepare herself for the eventuality, so she will *not* see herself as a failure should her baby be so delivered.

My own personal experience has been of c-section births. My first baby was delivered by emergency c-section after I had begun to lose blood (from a partial separation of the placenta), my waters had broken, and I had been in transitional labor for four hours. Doctors were staring at the monitor, orders were given, and I was hurried away to the operating room. Afterward, I think I can honestly say I felt no sense of loss at not delivering "naturally"; no sense of failure as a woman. All I felt was thanks and gratitude to be alive and well.

Lying there, through the pains of labor, my heart had gone out to women in the past, to all those women who had travailed in agony, often for days, only to die in childbirth. My baby had become trapped in the uterus, the doctor later informed me. Very likely she would never have emerged naturally through the birth canal. I am perhaps unusual these days, but I have a healthy respect for technology in medicine, for intervention that saves lives of both mothers and babies. My own level of success or failure did not even come into question. When it was time for the second birth, and the same doctor advised an elective c-section, as there was only a twenty-two-month gap, I accepted his decision. The second time, we know what the surgery entails; we also know what the risks and chances of labor entail.

Still, disappointment after a c-section is very common. Judy R. was in her late twenties, an executive secretary who was already back at work with a year-old baby when we talked. Judy's postpartum problems had been compounded by difficulties nursing her son because it hurt her breasts unbearably. She could see, looking back, that the two things worked together against her. "These days an inability to nurse is seen as a lack of real desire.

And the fact I had a c-section also made me look a failure, in my own eyes. My mother came to help after the birth but she only contributed further to my lack of confidence and depression. It was getting back to work that finally cleared the PPD. I was so happy to be doing something I knew I *could* do!"

Carol and Derek C. had also both attended natural childbirth classes. They had planned for Derek to be at the delivery, so the emergency c-section came as a great disappointment to the twenty-five-year-old couple. "I just felt a complete failure since I couldn't deliver naturally. I was angry at my body for letting me down," recalled Carol. PPD in the first months after her baby's birth was worsened by the shock of that enormous lifestyle change to Derek and her. "To say the least, I was overwhelmed by parenthood!" she exclaimed.

Kathy S. noted that comments other people make to c-section mothers may intensify the sense of failure, imposing those pressures of perfection on them. A friend had said to her, confidingly, "You poor thing, you'll never know what it's like to have a baby"; a night nurse had breezed through the ward, where two thirds of the women had just had c-sections, muttering, "Can't you mothers remember how to have babies any more?"

DEPRESSION IN PREGNANCY

Depression felt after a birth may in fact have begun during the pregnancy itself. The first trimester (one to twelve weeks) is noted for the metabolic changes that leave us with nausea, tiredness, and very often feeling down or mildly depressed. Less and less are accidental and unwanted pregnancies a cause of depression, as the majority of births these days are very much wanted. Nevertheless, the timing can sometimes be wrong in our lives. Pregnancy might come too soon in a marriage disrupting the ecstasy of a new relationship, or we may conceive sooner than we imagined and feel we had no time to prepare ourselves emotionally for the change of life.

Prepartum depression is not discussed professionally because obstetricians are used to the moods swings of the nine months. Dr. Katharina Dalton, however, has some significant comments on this period. She points out that some women do not receive enough progesterone late in their pregnancies, and experience depression similar to that of PMS or PPD. Instead of the elation and euphoria commonly experienced in the middle months, they feel terrible, suffering headaches and general malaise. She would prescribe progesterone in such cases, even in pregnancy (see pp. 49–50).

Doctors are quick to assume that women who have psychosomatic complaints and lack of energy and enthusiasm during pregnancy may be the ones to suffer PPD when, in fact, they may be the ones *not* to. Current research is looking into the relationship between mood and emotional changes in pregnancy and mood shifts after birth.

Previous abortions or several miscarriages before a healthy birth might also help contribute to PPD, either because the woman's self-image is loaded with a vision of these previous "failures," or because she is carrying too great an emotional investment in motherhood (implicitly in its "perfection"). Drs. R. Kumar and K. Robson, of the Institute of Psychiatry in London, have related symptoms of PPD to suppressed mourning, or guilt, over a voluntarily lost fetus.[30] The way we cope with therapeutic abortions these days, they emphasized; accentuates the ambivalence women might feel toward motherhood.

It is not easy to decide to abort. It is not easy to be a mother. Women's emotions are complex on both subjects. Perhaps some form of group counseling or therapy in abortion clinics might help women come to terms with their ambivalence and fears about motherhood *before* they finally take the plunge and become mothers.[31]

Some pregnancies are so difficult that we hardly feel surprised when the mother becomes depressed. Just think what she had to go through to have this baby, we say to ourselves. Jackie P. had been married eight years to Ben, and they were financially secure enough for her to give up working when, at age twenty-nine, she decided it was time for them to begin a family. After four years of trying to conceive and four miscarriages, Jackie conceived again and once again appeared to miscarry. An ultrasound scan, however, showed she had lost one of fraternal twins and the pregnancy continued. But not without more drama.

At seven months, Jackie developed preeclampsia and was ordered total bedrest. At eight and a half months high blood pressure was diagnosed and an emergency c-section advised. Her son was delivered healthy, but she learned later that both only narrowly survived. Jackie then spent thirty-six hours in intensive care on anticonvulsive drugs.

Because the couple's new home was not yet finished, Jackie went back to her mother's house, and a nurse was hired to help out. Jackie fired the nurse after three weeks because of their conflicting views on baby care. There was some crying, some exhaustion, she noted, but PPD itself did not set in until she and Ben were ready to move into their new home. A considerate and thoughtful man, Ben had bought all the groceries and even, Jackie remarked, put toilet paper in the new bathrooms. Proudly he carried Jackie and the baby over the threshold to start their new life.

"What did I have to be depressed about? After all this time I had a healthy son, a loving husband, a good marriage, and we even had our dream home. I was the woman who had it *all.* But for the next three months I was in the pits of depression. I saw no one and asked no one's help. How could I?"

Slowly the clouds of depression lifted. Jackie came to some conclusions about the cause of her PPD. Previously she had had a fallopian tube and an ovary removed, and the resulting depression reminded her of PPD. She felt her condition was partly hormonal but, as she expressed it, mainly due to exhaustion, the emotional upheaval of the previous nine months, and lack of sleep. Many women, in fact, have guessed at the cause of their PPD, but have been unable to validate their instincts because of the lack of knowledge about the condition.

PREMATURITY OR DISABILITY

Any mother can identify with the parents of a baby born prematurely or with some disability. Whatever feelings are experienced by the parents of a normal or healthy newborn can only be exaggerated by the very real stress of coming to terms with fear for the child's life, emotional deprivation if they cannot hold the baby, or anxiety about their family's future.

When she was seven months pregnant, bleeding heavily, twenty-three-year-old Sarah J. was ordered bedrest, but the bleeding continued and she had to be rushed to the hospital. The delivery was frightening, with a crowd of doctors waiting in the corridor who raced out of the room with her infant son, the moment he was born, to give him oxygen. One of his lungs had not inflated and he was moved to a downtown hospital with a neonatal intensive care unit. Sarah begged to be allowed home after thirty-six hours, finding it too miserable being with all the happy mothers.

When Sarah visited her son she was totally unprepared for the emotional shock. He was wired to tubes and machines, lying pathetically in a plastic box with portholes, pads on his eyes to protect him from the bright lights. There was further panic when a neurosurgeon was called in. But Peter was fine and recovered fast. After ten days he was moved back to their local hospital, where he was kept for six more days.

"It was the sixteenth day and my birthday," said Sarah. "I really hoped to take him home, but they insisted on keeping him one more day. That's when my blues set in. My husband was working nights, so I was home alone in the house. My father had died some twelve months beforehand. My husband and I went to the restaurant by the hospital to order a sandwich and the waitress got mine wrong. All this and now a dumb sandwich! I started crying and crying. She must never have had such a reaction to a sandwich before!"

For Sarah, the birth of Peter had been the most difficult experience of her life. She felt a relief now on expressing all those complex emotions. "How can you forget the pain, the joy, and the love involved in the birth of a child? The baby blues to me was just part of the *whole.*" Sarah was lucky. The blues for her was transitory, Peter recovered quickly, the nightmare was short-lived.

This letter came from a mother of two brain-injured sons. Shirley B., now in her late thirties, wrote, "I hope you will not neglect the topic, as so many do, of postpartum depression that occurs upon learning your child is handicapped. PPD is not only a normal reaction to a normal child."

Shirley's eldest son, now sixteen, was born severely retarded with autistic symptoms. The problem was not noticed at birth, but Shirley suspected something was wrong when, at five weeks, she felt he was hypersensitive. Left alone to deal with his handicap and her own disappointment, fatigue, and sense of failure, Shirley once begged a doctor to help her. "What can I do?" she cried. "Get rid of what is bothering you," the not so well-meaning doctor replied. Only years later did she dare go back and confront this man with what he had said in that time of grief. "I only meant you should get rid of the problems your son causes," was his flippant reply. Shirley sighed, "Oh, if only it were so simple. Wouldn't we be wealthy if we knew how to do that?"

Three years later, Shirley gave birth to another son. The family now knows that he has a milder form of the same autism, but thankfully he is bright and a reasonably normal child. Shirley has been told that the autism is caused by chromosomal damage that, in her case, is hereditary, for her brother was also born retarded. If she were going through pregnancy today, the obstetrician should take that history of retardation in her family as an indication for genetic counseling before she ever began a family.

Shirley's story highlights so much that is missing in our society: mainly, perhaps, the lack of any one professional to deal with the postpartum period, to help mothers cope with even the *normal* problems of parenting—fear, isolation, sense of inadequacy, responsibility—let alone the extra burdens imposed on the parent of a handicapped child.

Guilt and feelings of failure, which might normally lead to PPD for these parents, are added to the very real emotional, social, and even financial pressures of dealing with any handicap. These parents experience a sense of mourning for the perfect child they had dreamed of, for the perfect mother, or parent, they had fantasized. Shirley's experience was sixteen years ago. Today's parents discovering a handicap or mental impairment would, I hope, be offered basic societal help, would be able to turn to a group of parents with similar circumstances for support and guidance. Certainly no one should be left to the total despair and humiliation of begging a disinterested doctor for help and being told to get rid of the problem.

AFTER LAMAZE

What about society's views of mothers *after* the birth? "The baby-care books tell you when to bathe and burp, but not what to do when you're sitting there nursing, tears rolling down your face, or putting your child in its crib to cry it out because you can't handle it any more, or wishing you'd never had a child. They don't tell you what to do when you get home—after Lamaze," said Sharon W.

Is there really a way we can extend our knowledge of PPD, so we improve not only care and treatment at professional levels, but also the general information taught or available to pregnant women and new mothers? We take our pregnancies so seriously these days. We approach labor and delivery, and hospital and doctor management, like educated consumers. Lamaze, or some other childbirth education class, is seen as part of a normal premotherhood experience. We expect and demand the best of our bodies, of our professional health-care team, and of our ultimate relationship with the baby. Yet we are chronically guilty of the new myths of motherhood prevalent in our society. We never for a minute expect anything *should* follow after Lamaze.

We love the image of ourselves, as seen in the commercials and magazines: either the ethereal, beautiful, tender, nurturing mother, cradling her beautiful baby; or that other popular image today of the striding, smiling, self-confident, competent mother, skiing, running, cheerfully encountering the world, her baby in a Snugli or backpack. Being a mother can make for such pretty pictures.

Of course we like to think of ourselves that way: the fantasized image of ourselves as mothers is an integral part of the PPD perspective.

"I think it is a crime that all this emphasis and education is placed on childbirth and nothing is done to help a woman cope postpartum," said Jenny T. vehemently. A recent correspondent told me that the nurse in her hospital-run preparation class maintained that "no one gets the baby blues any more—it's a thing of the past." There would appear to be deep layers in the national psyche effectively blocking any move for change beyond the myths of motherhood.

Nancy E. telephoned me, as the result of several long talks, to relate the latest in the chain of events regarding her own PPD. Living in a small rural town, Nancy had not met anyone in the community who had also suffered. But she was willing to help others by talking, listening, or running groups and was anxious to start something going along those lines. First Nancy had broached the idea of setting up a postpartum group to her obstetrician and pediatrician. Neither felt there was a need, as no woman had ever asked for such meetings. She insisted, however, that both doctors put her name on file and that they put my magazine article in the same file, in case any depressed woman should ever come to them in the future.

Then she tackled her local childbirth education group, which was run by a social worker and a nurse. The social worker liked the idea of mentioning PPD, its causes and treatments, in the Lamaze classes. But the nurse, who had suffered some mild PPD herself, felt it would unduly worry or frighten the pregnant women and was not suitable for prenatal classes.

"Surely," said Nancy, "they could say that this might happen, and why, and that if it does this is someone to phone?" I agree with Nancy that such simple measures are a must. As one woman who had had severe PPD put it to me, "My baby was actually in danger from me. Yet I had no idea what was going on, that I could turn to anyone, or what to do. That sort of situation must stop."

Many pregnant women would rather *not* know about PPD, would prefer not to focus on any negative image of their future role. There is a fundamental optimism about a chosen pregnancy, a wonder in the magic and mystery of life, an overflowing excitement in the thrill of creating a life, of blending ourselves with a loved partner in one harmonious being. Maybe, biologically, we are tuned toward optimism, away from any negative thoughts. Perhaps, indeed, the pregnant woman can never be the target of education on PPD.

The question remains, who can the new mother turn to for help? If her obstetrician or pediatrician seems unwilling to deal with her personal problems, does that leave her with only the choice of mental health clinic, psychotherapist, or psychiatrist? Very often, one of the main problems experienced by a new mother is lack of anyone to confide in, someone to offer advice and maybe some reassurance. Very often, when women have turned to well-meaning advisers for help, maybe to their mother, family doctor, obstetrician, or even a priest, they have been fended off with a cheery "It's just one of those things," "no one dies of it," "you'll be fine, it's quite normal," or "get yourself out of the house and snap out of it."

We should not even expect help from the usual sources. Our own mothers might appear downright hostile to any mention of PPD if their history included denial of symptoms. Husbands may be scared and no doubt undergoing their own form of depression, leaving them with scant emotional resources to cope with a wife's moods, too. One woman's family priest told her she should battle against her selfishness.

HOW WE CAN HELP OTHER MOTHERS

Psychological or emotional disorders are among the least understood problems in society, despite their prevalence. Very few of us know how to deal with someone who is depressed, nor do we even want to. We have probably all been guilty of bad listening. If a new mother does try to unload her fears on our shoulders, what, if anything, should we do to help her?

The first piece of advice is that to deny the problem or try to cheer her up, which often seems the best course of action, will probably make her feel worse. Psychotherapist Judith Klein, who has a New York practice and a particular interest in women going through PPD (she is in her mid-thirties and the mother of a toddler and baby herself), explained that the implication behind saying "look on the bright side" is that the problem is within her, or that she is in the wrong.[32]

Laura S. experienced that kind of approach and it certainly made her feel worse. "It's such a difficult thing to talk about. I mentioned my depression casually once to my mother, but she never opened up about it. My grandmother and mother, all they lived for was children, how could she ever talk about such a *terrible* thing, was the impression I got." The only colleague Laura knew who was also having a baby seemed to be coping wonderfully and had a fat contented baby to show for it. Neighbors all were smiling and cheerful. It was obvious to Laura that the only person not happy as a mother was *Laura.*

Nancy E. finally saw a psychiatrist when her PPD became so disruptive to family life that her husband made the appointment. The psychiatrist gave her a course of antidepressant medication and offered support in educating her family about the biochemical causes of depression, which were not, he emphasized, Nancy's fault. But he said nothing to Nancy about any postpartum link.

Nancy also commented that her pediatrician, who was so closely involved with them in this period because of her problems with lack of milk supply and struggle to continue breastfeeding, showed total lack of sympathy with her problems. He disapproved of her taking the antidepressant medication and said frankly he would be pleased when she came off it. "I wasn't living up to his expectations of *me.* I was a mother and I shouldn't be on medication. My husband didn't like the fact I was taking antidepressants either, nor did my parents. My friends were critical, or caustic, or changed the subject whenever I brought it up. If they were embarrassed then I felt embarrassed. I used to feel I was a drug addict taking the pills."

Women friends, usually such a source of solace and support in our times of crisis, may react, seemingly out of character, with hostility toward a PPD mother. Presumably the new mother's emotional response contradicts some notion that the friend had about perfect motherhood; the friend may have undergone miscarriages or abortions; have experienced problems finding a man to marry and father her own children; or suffered infertility for months or years.

There are many reasons why women friends can resent a

mother's depression. But an understanding of our friends' hostility is hardly what *we* want to be feeling at this critical time. Somehow the lines of communication even between women have to be opened, certain old-fashioned barricades have to be broken down. A new mother may find a male friend more supportive in her crisis than a female friend.

Most women retire into their shells when they discover no one knows or cares to hear what they are talking about. "Thirteen years ago, I had my only child and suffered a terrible PPD. I have never discussed this with anyone at all," wrote a forty-three-year-old woman. Another correspondent, grateful to get her guilty secret off her chest, said, "Unknown to friends or family I've been in therapy since my son was five months old."

Parent support groups and mothers' discussion groups, which are flourishing in many towns and cities across the nation, are perhaps going to be the single most beneficial area of growth in helping mothers find other mothers to talk to, helping them through PPD. The groups of mothers with similar-age children (often evening groups are available for working mothers) meet to discuss problems of childcare and baby management and to explore the emotional and social changes of motherhood . . . the journey all must take to find that lost self.

Chapter 7

WHEN LOVERS BECOME PARENTS

When a couple become parents they are setting out on a totally different voyage from that of their prechild relationship. They are going to suffer not the pangs of the narcissist, but the very real pain of facing heavy and seemingly overwhelming responsibility; of strain and separation in their own love or erotic relationship; changes in their sexuality and libido; new awareness of what being female or male actually means.

Recently I was talking to Eleanor C. an as yet childless married friend in her early thirties, who whispered to me she felt the time was close when she and her husband would take the plunge. When I asked Eleanor whether she would continue working once she became a mother, and how would they pay for child-care, she became irritated and remonstrated, "Oh, come on. I just want a little baby."

We all "just wanted a little baby," didn't we? What we did not necessarily want was the person we became as a mother. An insurance office manager, 29-year-old Juliet T., said, "Nothing in the world could have prepared me for parenthood. I was euphoric about having the baby until I came home, and then I was overtaken by fear, anxiety, and deep sadness about my new responsibilities, by the enormity of what had just occurred, and by my passage into a new role."

Nina S. was even more explicit on this point. At thirty, a secretary for many years, single and living with Colin, who is the father of their child, Nina did not plan the pregnancy, but when it happened she realized she wanted a child. Colin agreed that the time was right, and quickly they became wrapped up in preparing for their new lives. Nina found the ensuing PPD an unwelcome shock, but she was able to see some of the disturbing forces in her life. "I had been used to doing exactly as I pleased for the first thirty years of my life. Now, suddenly, I didn't have as much as five minutes to myself, to take a long luxurious bath, to go out for a ride, even the simple pleasure of reading an article in a magazine had become something of the past."

Nina found herself wondering whether having the baby had all been a terrible mistake. Another mother put it even more bluntly: "I think many of us don't really enjoy being parents. We feel incompetent, we feel guilty, we feel trapped by it. Yet we can't admit it to ourselves."

The life stress scale of the social psychologists, which assigns scores to life crises (death of a loved one ranks highest and marriage often is next highest), has for some reason overlooked childbirth as a major stressor. George Brown and Tirril Harris, in their book *The Social Origins of Depression*, have analyzed the effect of social events on our ability to cope, adapt, or ultimately fall victim to depression. The authors conclude that our ability to adapt to stresses is mostly affected by "recent provoking factors" and "current vulnerability factors": if you lost your mother by the age of eleven, or if you have recently lost someone very close, your provoking, or vulnerability, factors would be very strong.[33]

My feeling is that childbirth is an enormous life stress, when linked to the desires, dreams, and expectations that brought us to want a baby in the first place. The craving to have a baby comes from a deep biological fountain of good will, a desire to nurture, sexual longings not consciously felt and a genetically programmed need for the human race to reproduce. These motivations often bear little relation to our ability to perform as wonderful mothers (or fathers), to deal with an infant, raise a toddler, or cope with an adolescent. "I just want a little baby," we say.

FINDING TIME FOR A CHANGING MARRIAGE

The baby-care books tend to trivialize the strains having a child can put on a marriage: they advise patience, understanding, supportive behavior, and an attempt to appreciate what the other partner is going through. This good advice may make us feel that if it's that simple, surely only *our* marriage is suffering. Everyone else out there is sharing baby care, having meaningful conversations in the evenings, smiling benignly over the sleeping infant in the crib, and then going off to bed to have erotic, romantic sex.

Jane Honikman, a mother from Santa Barbara, California, several years ago helped form PEP (Postpartum Education for Parents), one of the many invaluable parent support groups now available across the nation. Also coauthor of PEP's *A Volunteer's Reference Guide*, she is adamant that many new parents end up divorcing simply because they cannot cope with the overwhelming changes.[34] "The intimacy goes from their marriage, they lose interest in each other, all the energy goes into the children and there is no focus on the couple. At some point we have to stop and say, 'Why do we exist as a family?' and hope to save that marriage before it dissolves beyond repair."

Many marriages that were founded on unwritten principles of equality and sharing often relapse, once there is a baby, into traditional role-playing unions. Despite rhetoric on what men or women should or should not do in the house, I believe it is very difficult for husband and wife (with a baby) to dissociate themselves from those traditional roles. The woman sees herself as mother and housewife and her husband as "breadwinner." The man sees himself as father and money earner and his wife as "mother"; She is resentful that the whole burden of domestic duties and baby care is suddenly dumped on her. He is resentful that the whole burden of supporting this family falls on him.

Heather D. was a former teacher and part-time painter when she and her husband Eric changed from being a couple in their early thirties with few cares or concerns, other than the maximum enjoyment of their lives and each other, to being parents. Heather gave up her teaching job, believing she would now fulfill her creative ambitions while being at home with her family. But disenchantment quickly crept into the marriage.

"Eric would come home and find me watching TV a lot, or talking on the phone. The baby would be screaming. He'd yell at me for not cleaning the house and for doing nothing all day! I resented him fiercely for not helping out. I can tell you I threw dishes at the walls I was so mad. He never ever thought to criticize me for not cleaning the house *before* we had a baby. Why did it suddenly become my chore? You get to know a different side of your husband you don't necessarily like."

On both sides resentment can rear its ugly head. The man and woman withdraw into separate corners. It may take a lot of patience, hard work, and determination to keep a marriage afloat. Julia F., for example, was the kind of traditional woman who was happily married, content in her work and in their lovely home that she enjoyed keeping tidy. When their baby was due, twenty-nine-year-old Julia imagined she would give birth and then slip right back into her work and old routines. She certainly never imagined a marriage problem. At first Julia was proud to be up early cleaning the house, putting in the laundry, preparing the evening meal in her Crockpot, so her husband, Neil, could still have those delicious meals he was used to. She was energetic, enthusiastic, and glowing with pride in her ability to "have it all."

Then depression set in. For the first time in her life, she could not discuss her feelings with Neil. "Sometimes I felt like my whole life, physical and emotional, had changed, yet here he was still going to work in the morning, and coming home in the evening. It didn't seem fair that his adjustment to all this was minimal compared to mine."

Julia finally had to accept the fact that she was overwhelmed. She saw a doctor, who prescribed antidepressants, but they did not make her feel any better, just more tired and confused. She and Neil began to see a marriage counselor "because we don't want to lose our special relationship and we feel that talking to someone about the adjustment would be a help. We've been married three years and knew each other for seven years before that. We've had time to play, travel, and work; we know each other quite well, and hopefully we'll get through this." If only we could all be as wise and far-seeing.

A maternity nurse wrote to me about a near disaster in her marriage, with an eleventh-hour rescue. For Patty and Ted D. the problem was compounded by his work problems. Ted, who also was a nurse, doing many double shifts because of hospital understaffing and their own financial needs, felt trapped in a job he did not like. Patty, twenty-five years old, with two babies twenty-three months apart, missed her job and envied him for at least getting out of the house and being with other people. She had loved her job, but she felt she also loved babies. Now she was suffering a sense of desertion with Ted out of the house so much. "I was lonely, drained, and oppressed. I missed associating with friends at work. Ted had no idea how hard it was to be home with two little kids and what felt like no purpose in life. He thought it was a vacation for me!"

From his side, there was the desire to escape and have time to himself. When he came home he would want to go out hiking or fishing. Patty wanted him home to help her do the dishes, change diapers, take the kids out, wash the clothes. "I was so sunk in frustration and self-pity I could not hear my husband trying to tell me how frustrated he was in the job, which didn't pay what he deserved. He was feeling so sorry for himself that he had to support and maintain a family instead of being able to go out and play in the mountains, that he couldn't bear my unhappiness either."

Patty and Ted separated for one week. She says the split-up led to their mutual discovery "that we loved each other more than our respective miseries." After much talking, they agreed to move closer to their families, cooperate, and make time for each other.

We've all read the advice, countless times, in books and magazines: to talk with our partners, communicate, air our grievances, negotiate rather than fight, make space for adult loving. But when you're sunk in the pits of despair, hopeless and frustrated, it can be hard to find the energy or motivation even to talk.

Nina S. reminisced nostalgically: "I was used to spending unlimited time with Colin on weekends and evenings, just lying in bed, enjoying each other's conversation and bodies. The baby suddenly took up even the closeness we once had. Now it was all baby time, so when I went to bed, I more or less collapsed from fatigue. Colin was having many of the same feelings, I could tell, even though he didn't speak about it often."

A baby too soon in the marriage can lead to disappointment in the loss of romance and that early all-consuming form of love. The adaptation then is twofold: to a different form of marriage and to life as a threesome. Ginny W., at age twenty-seven, had been married only six weeks when she conceived. Ginny said that after the baby came, "I would end up crying to Rob that I wanted it to be like it was before. Just the two of us. I felt the baby was an intruder. My husband's stomach was in knots too. I was not the only one affected by this change."

In *Parenthood: Its Psychology and Psychopathology,* Therese Benedek asks why psychoanalysts have failed to study the developmental situation of parents.[35] Why have they focused all their studies on the development of children? She maintains that they failed to take an objective overview of the various stages parents go through for the simple reason that they are parents themselves and never thought about it![36]

The struggle for growth, the change from being a single unit, from being a child-adult without responsibilities, to becoming a parent with ultimate responsibilities, limitations, and conflicting emotions is a vital part of growing up.

WILL SEX AFTER CHILDBIRTH EVER BE THE SAME?

In the meantime, some of us are left wondering whether our sex lives will ever return to the excitement, romance, and eroticism of before parenthood. In baby-care books, sex after birth receives scant mention. Perhaps parents are not really supposed to be erotic people, for the implication is that the sexual urge is one we should *gladly* repress in our delight over becoming parents. What references are made tend either to be upbeat and blindly optimistic (everything should be back to normal in a few weeks, so just hang in there) or detailed. A Masters and Johnson study, for example, has discovered a lower level of sexuality even at three months postpartum and that achieving orgasm after birth can be more difficult because of fatigue or tension, because of breast tenderness, soreness after an episiotomy, exhaustion from c-section delivery, or fears that sexual organs have changed and that vaginal muscles are either tighter or looser.

One detail that has been overlooked is that a very real symptom of PPD is loss of libido. When that normal postpartum fall in thyroid occurs, it drops below the prepregnancy level and stays there for many months. Loss of thyroid seems to affect the female sexual response in a very direct way. For example, those on thyroid medication usually find a return to normal sexual response in two to three weeks.

Very little is said about deeper psychological strains from changing marital relationships, altered sense of identity, and variable moods. Such is the pressure on us to be having healthy (that is, continuous and frequent) sex lives that we dare not own up to abstinence. Where once we might have been ashamed to mention *having* sex, now we are ashamed to mention *not having* sex![37] What if we are experiencing no sexual desire after the six-week checkup with our obstetrician? Or, as one woman described, what can we make of no feeling in the vaginal area for up to eight months? What if our husbands seem to have turned off sexually? We are left floundering in fear about our own sexual viability.

Sex, as is always the case, is likely to be an indicator of other changes taking place within our psyches and within our relationships. Think again about the resentment a woman may feel toward her husband when he appears to have all the freedom, compared to her sense of entrapment, after the birth of their much-wanted child. She is feeling that her life has radically changed, while his remains pretty much the same in her eyes. Add to that the conflicts taking place at the core of their partnership and there are grounds for discontent on both sides.

Marital tension shoots to the surface; at best, this period of silence and withdrawal may give both parties time to absorb the impact of parenthood on their lives.

The after-birth relationship between a man and a woman undergoes many shifts. The woman very likely mothered her husband to some degree before the baby's advent. Without a child she enjoyed nurturing and caring for her man. He thrived on being pampered and catered to, being number one to the woman who, in return, he adored, as he once adored his mother. But now, with a baby, his wife does not want to mother him. Worse, she even feels contempt for his need to be mothered, when she so obviously feels her own need to be cared for. To her mind, this man she married and so loved has regressed into a self-centered child.

We should consider too what makes a woman, or a man, feel sexy. Certainly not fatigue, loss of identity, feelings of entrapment, or loss of self-esteem. As has often been shown in recent literature, both men and women need fantasies—of idealized partners, idealized situations, or an idealized self—to feel sexual. Without a strong identity how can we fantasize?[38]

Our sexuality, up until motherhood, had been based on a number of variables. How we related to men in general, how we felt about how we looked and dressed had all been important. None of these variables remained the same after we left our childless lifestyle.

Dianne McL. felt the decline in her sexuality even while she was pregnant. When her baby was nearly two months old, she wrote in her journal, "I haven't had sex for six months already, and really I feel I've lost all interest." Just getting big and fat to begin with had altered her self-image. "I was used to being a size nine, wearing tight clothes. That was part of my identity. I could turn men on in skin-tight jeans, and I knew it and liked it. But now I wouldn't even know what to do to *feel* sexy."

Let us go one step further. Dianne admitted to me that she loved having her baby daughter in bed with her. She did not mind that her husband, Randy, had taken to sleeping on the couch. "One night recently he came back to the bedroom. But I didn't want him. I was happy in bed with my daughter. I was breast-feeding, and it felt so close, just me and her."

What new mother hasn't felt that twisting conflict of loyalties? The baby has become her lover, the husband is the intruder. If not, the baby would be the intruder. The new mother is caught either way. Naturally, cast in this role of outsider, many men feel hurt and withdraw either angrily or in silence.

Unfortunately, the sexual impasse set up by the new parents deepens as the husband, the victim of this particular scenario so out of his control, suffers a chronic sense of rejection, which, coupled with his own changing sense of himself on becoming a father, becomes just too much for him to deal with. His reaction may be intensified by a reawakening of the jealous resentment he felt as a boy at his mother's rejection. The new father may respond in denial or anger. Often his reaction is to leave the house for longer periods during the day. He might find solace in work, where society implies he should be devoting more of his energies now that their need for money is greater. He might find refuge in exercise, sports, afteroffice drinking, or, of course, as has so often been the case, in the arms of another woman.

The sexual withdrawal a woman experiences on becoming a mother should certainly be the focus of our interest, and not the center of denial. For some women even being caressed or the very thought of sexual penetration is like an invasion. At this very sensitive, vulnerable time, their sexual needs have transferred into a deep cry to be nurtured. That their husbands need them, are demanding of them, can just lead to their greater withdrawal. The new mother feels she is giving on all levels, all at once: emotionally, physically, spiritually; to the baby, to her other children, to her husband. Sex seems like the least pressing need at this time.

Psychotherapist Judith Klein offered some insights into why we might undergo this unexpected response to new motherhood. One of the reasons we mothers feel so sexually attached to our babies is that the experience of giving birth has reawakened the memory of our own birth and those infantile longings for our mother. We want to relive that cuddly, warm, perfect security; the joyous skin contact; the giving sort of sexuality, rather than the give and take of adult heterosexuality. Klein explained more about this relationship with our mother and how it can affect our marriage.

"One of the things therapists often have to deal with is a woman's apparent loss of interest in sex, or her marriage, when she becomes a parent. On the surface it may look as though the relationship is at fault, or that she is rejecting motherhood, but really this all goes much deeper.

"At age five or six she would have gone through the Oedipal stage, when as a little girl she fantasized having a baby with daddy. These fantasies made her feel tremendous guilt about the strong feelings she had for the parent of the opposite sex, and she learned to be afraid of her mother's retaliation: that she would be angry, resentful, jealous, or punishing. If her parents divorced at this time, that would have made things far worse, for it would have been as though mommy had said, 'Here, have daddy.'

"The Oedipal fantasy is repressed over the years, but is often reactivated by the birth of her own child. The undesired fantasy is so anxiety-provoking that she tends to retreat into a masochistic defense and turn against her husband, not allowing herself any pleasure from the relationship—by withdrawing sexually, or maybe having affairs, or deliberately provoking the breakup of the marriage."

Sexuality is linked generally to feelings of energy, psychological balance, and normal mental and biological functioning. It is not encouraged by a situation in which we are overloaded by emotional demands, feeling drained, empty, that there is not enough of us to go around. For some of us, marriage counseling may be the answer; for others, a weekend or evening away together, or simply setting aside time to talk. Somewhere, somehow, we have to find our sexuality again. We have to work at who needs nurturing (the answer probably is both partners), who has what to give.

Julia F., for example, feeling that her marriage to Neil had fallen into decay since the baby had come, decided to book a hotel room on Valentine's Day, fill it with champagne and candles, and take her husband there for dinner. "If I didn't make some kind of effort soon, I knew I would lose him. Even holding hands those days seemed like such an effort. There just wasn't enough of me to go around," she said.

WHEN SEPARATION SEEMS THE EASIER OPTION

Resentment, mutually felt, can reach such a climax that the marriage may begin to look irretrievable. Divorce then appears the much easier option. We don't really have to look at the statistics to know that parenthood drives many a couple finally apart. Maybe the couple has begun to see in each other a new, less flattering, image. Maybe the battle for power and control in the relationship has taken on such shifting demarcation lines that neither feels at ease with the situation. Being a mother may have given the woman a new-found sense of power, which could disturb the sensitive balance of power that kept the couple at peace. Maybe her sexual withdrawal (or his) has been the final wedge that sets them truly asunder. A lot of work needs to be done in a lot of marriages to right this situation. I wish more sympathy and understanding would be extended to the *couple* at such a crucial time.

Cheryl J. had a full-time job as an executive secretary. At twenty-eight, she found herself living alone with her year-old son, separated from her husband, Scott, who walked out on them when Billy was just four and a half months old. Theirs was not an uncommon scenario in today's world. Cheryl had become aware, after Billy arrived, that Scott wanted to be mothered and that she did not want to mother him. She resented his not helping her in the house, and she resented that she *had* to work because of their family's financial situation, and consequently could not be the kind of mother she had always imagined herself.

"I would raise hell with Scott, that I could not do everything. I was back at work, coming home to household chores and mothering. Scott would leave the house for four and a half hours a night while I tried to catch up. I'd be asleep with the baby next to my bed and he wanted to know why I was always sleeping when he came home. I ended up trying to explain, crying, that I couldn't do it all. I needed help, if I was to continue working. Really, I wanted to stay home and raise my children. I wanted to be a good wife."

Cheryl believed her PPD was brought on far less by the separation than by her husband's bad adjustment to becoming a father. She could not, of course, see his side of the picture. Cheryl was resenting not being able to live out her ideal image of herself as a mother. She resented playing both mother and father (breadwinner and household domestic). She felt her depression ease when Scott left them. This way, at least, she regained all the control. "I ended up better off without him. In fact, my PPD ended when my husband left me."

Many women have suggested that men need sensitizing to the effects of PPD; that they should learn what is expected from them in the year after a baby's birth. These women want their men to know that a new mother needs mothering by her husband. They say a new mother would respond better to a man who is nurturing, supportive, patient, and undemanding. Men could understandably respond, "What about us? We need understanding too. What about our needs?"

Indeed, the suffering men may undergo in the process of becoming a parent is grossly overlooked. Maybe this is not surprising in a society that has only just begun to consider what women are undergoing. Nevertheless, when we consider the complex effects of the changes in men's lives brought on by childbirth, we should focus on them as much for the women's sake as for theirs.

Chapter 8

ON FATHERS AND SOME SPECIAL-CASE MOTHERS

If PPD is induced by a biochemical reaction to the act of childbirth, how, you might ask, can it be experienced by fathers, adoptive mothers, or stepmothers? (The other two sections in this chapter, on older mothers and single mothers, fit more easily into the accepted formula.) Yet new fathers, adoptive mothers, and stepmothers do, by their own description, suffer PPD.

Although I have tried hard to shift the blame from women themselves for the depressions they may suffer, my intention throughout Part Two has been to draw a much-magnified artist's impression of the feelings and emotions we may never recognize consciously but which, nonetheless, can affect us crucially on becoming parents. Taking the case first of fathers, the psychological impact of parenting may be just as overwhelming to them as to their wives.

The majority of men will not go into severe PPD, as would be experienced by a mother, because of the lack of the biochemical quotient. But the resulting confusion in the new father's mind, especially as he may be receiving little or no sympathy for his feelings, can lead to a chronic form of stress or depression that will not be resolved until years later and may be expressed in the abuse of alcohol or drugs, breaking up the marriage, or suffering a stress-related illness, such as a heart attack.

Paradoxically, though fathers are unlikely to receive much sympathy from society as a whole (it is still not seen as manly to be concerned about one's fathering), we are in the midst of a huge "joy of fatherhood" cultural media blitz. The ultimate effect of this emphasis may be to increase levels of PPD in men as they too scramble to achieve a preconceived view of perfection. A current bestseller on fathering, *Good Morning, Merry Sunshine,* by Bob Greene, may bring a smile of recognition and delight to those fathers who have already adopted some of the myths of the new man to their lives, who happily parade their newborns in Snuglis or backpacks around the parks or supermarkets.[39]

We are still left with far too many unanswered questions. There are the millions more men who have not taken on the mantle of new man, who do not wish to consider myths of new fatherhood. There are men who wish they could be "new fathers" but feel they fail before even beginning. There are men whose wives have seen in their spouses just that sort of image and, once they become parents, the wives are disappointed in their husbands' behavior.

We have not yet had time or distance to judge the impact on men of their new fathering, or its impact on our children, or on *ourselves,* now that we women have new levels of expectation with which to assess our husbands as partners. Major questions of control and power come into play between men and women when they become parents. Many women find it harder than they imagined to adjust to life with a new father, when that entails handing over many of the decisions about the child's life to the husband which, traditionally, had all been the woman's domain. The tired wife, complaining that her husband won't make up the bottles, get up in the night, or find a new baby-sitter when their regular help calls in sick, is the same wife who will not give her husband the space or the time to fulfill his part of the bargain.

The woman subtly takes the reins of control out of his hands because, in honesty, she feels insecure without that control. It is never easy to delegate; it is certainly hard to give up one area of dominance in the home and out of it, an area women have clung to for centuries. Many marriages are broken by just this pressure. The man is usually blamed ("He deserted her when they had a newborn—he just wasn't prepared to take on his responsibilities," we say in criticism), yet sometimes I wonder if such men are instead victims of ill-defined new roles.

Unable to comprehend what his place should be in this new family setup; not allowed his traditional role of provider, voice of authority and backup supporter; not allowed, in place of that, the new role of equal, sharing partner; finding himself undermined on all levels, he leaves. "At least divorced, with a reasonable custody arrangement, I get to see my son on my own terms. I get to make decisions and form my *own* relationship with him," commented Frank M., divorced father of a three-and-a-half year old. "She really took over the whole thing, and I was left out, pushed out, like a nobody." Frank left the family home when his son was four months old. Looking back, he realized that his desertion was a way of keeping some of that control he had so needed and wanted.

Nick, Laura S.'s husband, on talking about her still-current PPD five months after the birth of Bobby, said of course it was putting a terrible strain on their marriage, though they had been married for ten years. "You need an awful lot of money in the emotional bank when you decide to have a child," he added quietly, not wishing to get more deeply involved in the discussion.

When men become fathers they can become prey to the same psychological and emotional upheavals as their wives. The father may find old childhood conflicts reactivated, relive his own demands on his mother, or pass through unresolved conflicts with his father, which can be manifested in sexual withdrawal from his wife. If a man had problems relating to, identifying with, or feeling loved by his father, the passage into fatherhood may make him fear confrontation with these sides of himself.

A new father may suffer sibling rivalry with the baby over his wife's attention and love. The rivalry will emerge in an unwelcome resentment toward the baby, who, he feels, does not love him. Or the baby's crying, and obvious preference for its mother, can bring back fears of not being loved in his own infancy.

Sexually, the new father may have begun to discover confused signals in himself once his wife became pregnant. Whether her libido was directly affected or not, his might have been. Oedipal longings for his mother reemerge in a form of terror or revulsion toward his wife in the pregnant state.

Then, too, if his wife suffers PPD, the new father may be called on to play a much stronger and more supportive role than he ever expected, as Kathy S.'s husband, Bill, had to. Bill coped wonderfully, but this unexpected demand on a new father can lead to his own breakdown, as, confused, he is left wondering what happened to his wife, to his fantasies of her as a mother, to his fantasy of family life. Suffering his own identity crisis, fearing his life has gone out of control forever, feeling just as trapped as she is, the father may react in a similarly depressed fashion, or his response may be to withdraw more obviously from the home and bury himself in work.

As Judith Klein points out, we have always attributed men's moods to other stresses: pressure at work, desire to make more money to support their family, fear that their wife's devotion to the baby is leaving them out in the cold. Men are just learning to open up and talk about their feelings, so perhaps in the near future we will begin to hear a lot more about fatherhood and its impact on men.[40]

The pioneer men, who have reversed roles with their wives and acted as househusbands, or really shared equally in the child-care, could have important messages from the front. Simon S. was twenty-eight years old when he and Dana had their daughter, Estelle. Dana already had a good job as a magazine editor, a seemingly flourishing career that could easily support them both. Simon was not as strongly attached to his job, and, as he had always wanted more time to develop his writing and musical pursuits, he agreed to stay home with the baby, at least for the first year.

Such are society's pressures and needs for the image of happy "new fathers" that Simon has often been quoted in upbeat magazine articles and on television as an exemplar. I have known

Simon and Dana for many years. Although I did not really understand what was happening to them at the time, I used to sum up Simon's depression and black moods as "housewife's blues" in those early years of his retreat into the home.

They had moved to a pleasant leafy suburb, an easy commute for Dana from the city. Simon enjoyed the peace and the quiet routine, but inevitably he became isolated and withdrawn. He would chat with mothers in the park and at the supermarket, but no real friendships developed. "How could they?" Simon joked. "I'd have all those husbands banging on my door." Simon was busy projecting his own self-image of the new myth. Of course he was happy, he was out of the rat race, he didn't have to commute, and Estelle was a charmer. But his writing did not progress and his moods became very black.

To make matters worse, Dana's career took a sudden upward leap. She changed jobs twice, was recruited by a television network, and ended up as a minor celebrity, with appearances on television talk shows and a magazine column under her own name. To ease Simon's despair, she hired a part-time housekeeper, giving him more freedom. Simon was hospitalized for depression before he received a foreign assignment to write a long article, and with relish he took his pen and notebook and vanished for six weeks.

Simon reemerged sane and wise. He did not want to return to the working world, and that was a major problem he had to work out for himself. He needed time and self-confidence to push himself as a writer, and that meant his earning power was limited, to say the least. What happened to Simon is what happens to so many women once they become mothers. Torn from their former lifestyle, they suffer a sudden identity crisis, loss of self-esteem, and loss of freedom. For Simon the deep questions must have been: Was he man or woman? Was he nurturer or provider? What did masculinity mean to him and to the outside world? Dana confessed that she finally came to the realization that she had to pay a housekeeper, as Simon would never do all the work of a housewife. He would not clean the house, cook the meals, and do the laundry each day. Intent on keeping her own motherhood image intact, Dana worked herself to the bone, cooking for the family every evening, and even preparing Simon's lunch for the next day. What working husband ever does that for his wife?

Dana also noted that they have sought help from marriage counseling at least three times in the last eight years. They have both taken the time and made the effort to work at what has proved to be a very successful marriage and an interesting supportive partnership.

When roles are reversed, we are more sensitive to the vulnerable and precarious balance that keeps a relationship alive and both partners sexually and emotionally content. We do not offer such sensitivity to the average traditional relationship, where the wife assumes those roles that were so burdensome to Simon.

One way to alleviate their problems, Dana discovered, was to make sure their finances were more equal. The fact that the house was repaired, the new car bought, the vacation taken when Dana's bank account was large enough, only worsened Simon's low self-image. In a classic image of real role reversal, Dana decided to support Simon more completely. She channels monthly income into *his* bank account, balancing their equity. "We have a lot to learn yet, but I believe we have both been happier this way. And Estelle certainly has loved having her father around all these years," Dana commented.

There is a price we pay for motherhood or fatherhood, and that price is painfully clear when father plays mother. Still we refuse to see the strain and stress we expect women to live with when they become mothers. When a thirty-five-year-old father of a newborn was recently forced to give up working because his wife suffered a postpartum stroke and was left in a coma, medical insurance paid for nursing help to come to his house for part of the day so he could get to work or visit his wife in the hospital. A tragic situation and a caring insurance system. But would anyone think to offer that help to a new mother if her husband were hospitalized? No, women are expected to struggle on alone, without help or support. We just expect her to go about her business and not complain. "You wanted the baby, didn't you?" is said with a critical tone and resentful expression if a new mother dares to voice her exhaustion or inability to cope.

OLDER MOTHERS

Many people come to their parenting with a bagful of emotional investment in their ability to do it *better* than previous generations, friends, or colleagues, and they are convinced they can have it all. One group that has particular difficulties are the older mothers.

When I had my first baby, I was thirty-one years old and imagined I was part of the new "older mother" generation. Now I realize I was relatively young.

These mothers have invested much of their lives into their work, and, having a baby somewhere near the age of forty, they are determined to prove, along with their partners, that they are certainly as good, if not better, than the traditional or younger mother. Aware that they somehow offend society's beliefs that women past thirty or thirty-five are too old, that they run an increased risk of bearing a Down's syndrome baby, that they might be set in their ways, inflexible, or too tired, they have a *fierce* determination to succeed, to prove they are in fact little short of perfect. Their expectations may be even further removed from reality than younger mothers'.

Let us look at some of the deeper psychological difficulties inherent in late motherhood, or implicit in the delaying process, for these women have delayed having a baby for the major part of their reproductive lives. In her essay "Psychotherapy with Pregnant Women," therapist Joan Raphael-Leff notes that when a woman comes to motherhood later, pregnancy has been consciously set aside, avoided, ignored, maybe terminated, possibly ambivalently pursued, and denied throughout the preceding years. The conflicting emotions from those earlier years will still be in the subconscious even if consciously overcome.

Maybe the woman's delaying tactics were used until she met the right man or achieved a certain status at work. Maybe the ticking of the biological clock finally forced a decision. The excitement that can come with this abrupt change in viewpoint, with the welcome release of a long-repressed mothering instinct, with the overcoming of fear and denial, can be so heady, so all-consuming, that never for a minute will the older mother let a small negative voice whisper in her ear, "Watch out for reality!"

What is reality for older mothers? Biological clocks cannot be denied, and although having a baby can in some ways be rejuvenating (you feel the age of the traditional mother, somewhere in her twenties), there is no denying that tiredness, fatigue, and exhaustion are very much complements of this form of parenting.

Mary S., for example, is an exciting woman. A smart, breezy newspaper reporter with a string of books to her name, she has an enviable life with an attractive husband and an adorable fifteen-month-old son. Mary had just turned forty when we met. When I asked Mary if she suffered any PPD since Noah's birth, as I had noticed she never finished a sentence and often appeared totally distracted, she laughed easily. "When he was an infant, no. It's now that he is a toddler I cannot manage it. I really feel I'm on a treadmill, with work, and my writing projects, and looking after Noah.

"Bruce and I both really wanted this child. Now I'm forty and here I am with a lovely little boy. I'm remarkably grateful for the opportunity to have had him. I never imagined it would be possible for me. But I have been shocked to discover my own limitations as a parent. I just don't have the patience. There are times I feel I'm about to crack up. I wonder 'where's *me?*' "

Older mothers, and fathers, do tend to be more grateful to have had their children. They know how much a child has enriched their lives, perhaps improved their marriage, that not to have had a child would have been a terrible loss. They feel more guilt than the average parent in suggesting anything might be wrong. The efforts to deny impatience, fatigue, depression are stronger than for most of us. ("We told you it would be hard having a baby at forty," they hear tongues wagging in the background.)

When I talked to Mary, she refused to say anything at first that would affect the rosy picture she liked to promote. But once she trusted me, she talked more honestly. When I suggested to her, for example, that she might stop writing the books, if running her career with the newspaper, managing husband and child, plus having a social life was all proving too much, she stared at me, nonplussed. "I have to do the books. That's my only creative outlet. The newspaper job is mostly for our income. We couldn't get by on just one salary now, and anyway I like the structure it imposes on my life. But the books, writing, is my greatest love. And so is Noah. I can't cut either of them out of my life."

Then, sighing, she admitted, "I am just not the type to find it cute and funny when I'm trying to do a layout of pictures for a deadline the next day, on the dining room table, when Noah comes in for the third time and messes it all up. You know what I've been doing on Saturdays? While Noah naps, which is for about an hour and a half these days, I jump in a cab and race for the office, where I can snatch an hour or so of peace and quiet to get on with my work. It's worth the ten-dollar cab fare for my sanity!"

Many an older, or a working, mother understands why men escape into their work once they have a family. Given half a chance the women would do the same. Anything for peace, tranquility, and a feeling of being in control of one's life again.

Even if older mothers are not set in their ways, they are likely to be used to certain degrees of competence, control, independence, freedom, and to expect or demand areas of privacy and tranquility in their daily routine. The screaming bedlam of a house full of young children may be harder on their equilibrium than on a younger woman's. Broken sleep may affect them physically more strongly. It may be difficult to tolerate mess, chaos, and crisis, to be patient with a young child's interruptions and constant needs, which conflict with their own needs as a woman, wife, or worker. Whether that is an argument in favor of having children at a younger age, I very much doubt. It is something they should be aware of and accept.

Lily P., now in her early forties and back part-time at her job with a city housing program, had three boys when she was thirty-three, thirty-five, and thirty-seven. There were definite pluses on the side of being an older mother, she maintained, but the minuses should be watched out for. Basically Lily can see a need for one thing when dealing with young children—*energy.*

"By the time I was thirty-nine, with a two year old and two others under five, I was exhausted. It nearly drove my husband and me apart. I went weeping to a doctor several times and he gave me tranquilizers, which helped momentarily [she reported regaining sexual energy and fantasizing about younger men in the streets!]. But at one point I really just about cracked up.

"I have always expected, indeed demanded, to have help with the housework and to look after the children when they were little. I had to give up my job completely for two years, as I just couldn't cope. Even now I have only gone back two days a week —I'm lucky I can do that—because any more just puts me under a tremendous strain. The way of life has put a drain on our finances, but my husband has had to agree to it. It was a sacrifice we had to make as a couple, because I really do not have the energy necessary."

SINGLE MOTHERS

Single mothers may also fall into the trap of investing too much myth and optimism into their ability to cope, and consequently overlook some of the unconscious motivating forces that might lead them to distress and PPD. The single mother who chooses to become a parent without a partner, or husband, is almost bound to expect the best of herself and to deny many emotional problems she faces along the way. Other single mothers, who came to their position by default, because of an unwanted separation from the baby's father or his refusal to marry her at the last minute, may fail to connect their mood with the birth of the baby, imputing all their depression to the sense of desertion and betrayal. The baby is seen by these mothers as the one being who brings them happiness, who makes them feel loved and worthwhile, that their life is not altogether hopeless.

A single mother's anxiety and PPD therefore may not show itself in despair, but rather will emerge in her overprotectiveness. Not having anyone around to support her, she may find it hard to leave her baby with a sitter or in day care. As one single mother put it, "We chain ourselves to the source of our duress, like madwomen."

Overprotectiveness; chronic fear that the baby might die, from crib death, for example; inability to move the baby out of her bedroom or, in some cases, her bed; all tend to reflect the mother's own feelings of loneliness and being unloved and *her* fear of rejection, rather than the baby's.

Single mothers are expected to continue working and run up against little criticism for doing so. They are treated like fathers by our society and may be offered more help and support than would be offered to a traditional mother. The single mother's situation may be viewed by the outside world more accurately than that of other mothers.

Dr. Jessie Bernard noted that any woman, once a mother, knew what single motherhood was all about.[41] However helpful her husband, however supportive and financially sound, ultimately the responsibility for that child is hers. Eight or nine times out of ten it is she who is the one to get up at 3 A.M., bathe, feed, wipe the floor, arrange for the baby-sitter, hug, or take the day off work when the child is sick or needs to go to a birthday party.

ADOPTIVE MOTHERS

Adoptive mothers have not given birth. They cannot argue that hormonal shifts might have brought on the biochemical changes leading to depression. Yet women who adopt babies or small children are also subject to depression once the baby has joined their family.[42] There have been few statistics on the incidence of adoptive mothers suffering PPD, but statistics can only reflect the numbers of mothers who report such unwelcome feelings to a doctor or psychiatrist. How many adoptive mothers would report feeling depressed once they have the baby—the same baby they have fought long and hard to be given, with the subsequent fear that the agency might take the baby away again —when they and their husbands have spent months, or maybe years, convincing the social workers what normal, stable, secure people they are?

Adoptive mothers are subject to all the same frustrations and emotional overcharges as natural mothers, fathers, or any parents. They too will be shocked by the reality of motherhood, compared with their dreams and fantasized version. They will endure that sense of entrapment, the loss of identity, submersion of ego, and possibly feeling of despair that their decision has not been the right one. When an adoptive mother experiences such feelings, her guilt, shame, and anger at herself are likely to be even stronger than that of a natural mother because she has convinced herself, as well as the agency, that the one thing she wanted in the world was to be a mother.

Heavy emotional investment in the ideal of being a mother is therefore the adoptive mother's most immediate trigger for psychological distress, which can lead to depression. Her own negative self-image as a woman, which will have been cultivated over the years of her infertility or recurrent miscarriages, will also be playing its part. It is unlikely that any woman who has tried unsuccessfully, and with increasing desperation, over the years to conceive her own child, who has suffered the indignities and humiliations of infertility testing, who has had to accept that she and her husband will not be able to make their *own* baby (i.e., be normal parents) and that their only option is to adopt will avoid all the unconscious negative feelings about her femaleness and worthiness as a mother once she has a real child to look after.[43]

Perhaps the most typical kind of PPD (though, as PPD means postpartum depression, it can only be linked as a related syndrome, due to similar causes of psychological stress) experienced by an adoptive mother is that described by Georgette F. Her reaction was little different from that of many a natural mother, only her case was exaggerated by the speed with which she suddenly, in a matter of minutes, was thrown into motherhood, with no time for rehearsal or real preparedness.

There was building excitement beforehand, then the phone call to say they could bring the baby back home, and then *wham,* the reality—being a perfect mother was nothing like she had fantasized. At twenty-seven, a former data processing supervisor who had been in her job for nine years, Georgette received the phone call on a Wednesday evening that she and her husband, Bill, could pick up their adoptive baby in the middle of the next week. Georgette and Bill had been married for seven years, and had been trying to adopt a baby for the last three years. Now their dreams were about to come true.

Friday was her last day at work, and Georgette had it all planned that Monday through Wednesday would be spent cleaning the house, preparing herself to welcome little Zoe. On Monday, however, calling the caseworker to see if Zoe was well, she was told to come pick her up that day. Georgette went into a panic. Later that day, the house was full of party guests to greet Zoe into their lives. Then the door closed on an empty house, and Georgette began to learn what motherhood was really like. PPD set in as the last guest closed the door to the empty house, she recalled.

"Before the baby, Bill and I were used to being out of the house a lot. Of course I had always spent my days with other adults at work, holding adult conversations. All of a sudden it was so different! I couldn't take Zoe out because of the cold weather. I was imprisoned in my home with an eight-pound warden. I'd beg Bill in the evenings just to take the three of us to the grocery stores, never one of my favorite chores, but now it seemed like a wild excitement. Anything just to go for a ride in the car."

Georgette suffered enormous PPD and guilt for these feelings. After all that time convincing the agency they would be the best parents in the world, she wondered if they had misjudged themselves. That time rests vividly in her memory, but it did pass. Georgette and Bill now have two beautiful adopted daughters, and they escaped *none* of the psychological and situational side effects of becoming parents.

SECOND-HAND MOTHERHOOD

Becoming a stepmother means you take on parenting second-hand. The stepmother learns everything about parenting, with the negative aspects presented first. She is not in control, is often ill-regarded, and is an object of jealousy or resentment. The consequent guilt and anger may be a heavy burden. The psychological upheaval tends to be accentuated when the stepmother brings home her own baby, and the other children feel ousted from the nest.

Twenty-eight-year-old Lee G. maintained that the many ups and downs of her life, even the trauma of her own divorce, were never as bad as the PPD she experienced when, believing herself blissfully married to a second husband who also very much wanted to start a new family, she brought the baby home to her five-year-old stepson, Dan. Lee was elated that day. But because she had worked for eleven years as a legal assistant, the day her husband, Jeff, left her home with Dan and baby Louise, her world shattered. She was faced with a withdrawn, resentful, five year old who would not offer any love to Louise, and she had to deal with her own conflicting emotions over having wanted this baby and how she felt about being a real mother. "I felt cheated, frustrated, hurt, and most of all scared. Inadequate with my own baby, stupid, out of control and dreadfully alone." As Lee pointed out, "The problems of delivery were nothing compared to the emotional stress in the weeks that followed."

A thirty-five-year-old nurse, who had a fifteen-year-old son from a previous marriage plus a two year old and new baby from her second marriage, really believed all her dreams had come true. Said Sheila A., "I had wanted it all—husband, baby, home—so badly. Yet, when I gave up full-time work with the first baby, by the fourth month I had gone into a deep tailspin of despair. Then the second baby came along twenty months later, and I was floundering under stress, with too much to do and not enough outside stimulation."

For Sheila, the result of her emotional overload was total sexual withdrawal. She reported no vaginal feelings for over eight months. Sheila had, like so many special-case mothers, invested far too much in motherhood. Her first marriage, her first attempt at mothering (the now teenage son) were far from wonderful experiences. Now she had a second chance, and, feeling so grateful, she was doubly determined to live up to her ideals.

The reality of motherhood for Sheila, who was used to hospital life, was oppressive. Depressed, guilty, tied to the house, fatigued, Sheila finally admitted some truths to herself and returned to work. Getting away from motherhood, she confessed, had been her cure. With an active working life, an exercise class to help alleviate the stress, and her new, loving family, she learned to approach her mothering role more sensitively, more realistically, and less idealistically. Once the pressures were off, Sheila was able to feel happy again and her sexual feelings for the husband she loved so much returned.

Chapter 9

My Mother, My Baby, Myself

I wasn't prepared to accept the idea that our previous relationship with our mothers could have much relevance to postpartum mood until midway through my research. The whole idea sounded too involved, too critical of women, too redolent of stereotyped images of how women should be. "She's depressed because she rejected her mother"; "she has a hard time relating to her femininity"; "a tomboy with masculine identification, aggressive in work, controlling, refusing to accept her female role." I think we have a right to feel irritated by the assumption that there is only *one* type of normal behavior and that to react otherwise makes us abnormal or deviant.

Researching the book, meeting other women, talking to them, reading their letters, I became more confident myself, grateful to understand that PPD can affect any woman. The people I was in contact with were individuals. Some loved baking cookies and staying home, others had struggled up the corporate ladder and enjoyed a successful working life, most were somewhere in between. Seeing that PPD was no respecter of persons, I felt more willing to dig deeper into the complex tie of mother, daughter, and child.

Because research into PPD has for years been the domain of the psychiatric profession (if you recall, the view that PPD might have strong links with the physiological changes of childbirth, although first arrived at in the nineteenth century, disappeared from the professional eye until recently), by far the largest amount of literature available in professional journals is from the psychoanalysts. Without being frivolous, I recommend some of this literature as bizarre reading material and a perfect indicator of the state of public opinion on women over the past few decades.

The reason I had objected so strongly to comments in these academic articles that PPD no doubt related to a woman's relationship with her mother, or repudiation of her mother, had led me to scribble a message in the margin of one of my notebooks: "Surely we must all have a problem with the image we hold of our own mothers these days? If that's the case, do we now have a generation of PPD sufferers?"[44] I had in mind the revolution in thinking about women, and in the reality of women's lives, since the 1960s, and our current marked turn away from values of the past. Was this transitional crisis in the role of women then playing a larger part in our own acceptance of motherhood?

My research began, as so much does, in myself. I had to think long and hard about the image I held of my mother, the one that had so upset me when I felt associated with it in my own mind.

With my two babies, I was utterly depressed to realize that my lifestyle was not so revolutionary and different from my parents' and specifically my mother's life pattern. Even though part of me wanted to be a loving, caring, kind mother to my children, as she had been to my sister and me, the sense of becoming like her was terrifying and had dragged me down.

Over the years I have grown to understand that my rebellion against my mother was an attempt to break away from my desperate *need* for her, my dependence and dependent love. My mother and I are good friends, as adults, with a sympathy for our differences. It is through our mothers that we learn to judge, forecast, and assess ourselves as women in the world. The very act of becoming a mother seems to narrow our sense of choices, of ourselves as women, almost overnight, to a vision of ourselves in her light, as though a net had been mysteriously cast over us, reducing us all to *mother*.

Daughters do have to separate from their mothers, we now know. Failure to separate is an unhealthy psychological sign. Our own daughters will have to enact a similar rebellion even if, right now, we like to imagine they will be so inspired by our brilliant, struggling example that they will accept us just as we are without moments of rebellion. The emotional distress the psychological separation from our mothers induces may often contribute to PPD.

CONFLICT WITH THE MOTHERING ROLE

The deeper feelings of loss of a separate identity, independence, and self-esteem are all most likely linked to this new self-image, and we are exposed, as the psychiatrists say, to a conflict with the mothering role. Their interpretation of this conflict is what I object to.

Frederick Melges, then of the department of psychosomatic medicine at the University of Rochester School of Medicine and Dentistry, wrote an article in 1968 that, because it is now nearly twenty years old, is somewhat archaic in its views.[45] Melges let himself be trapped in traditional male views of what a woman's role or place in society should be. Thirty-five percent of the one hundred postpartum patients (he was looking for incidence of PPD) questioned had "played with dolls slightly if not at all," and "had not worked as baby-sitters" (thereby casting a future generation of sexually and socially liberated young girls into heavy PPD). Melges's respondents expressed a preference to be men, said they related more to their fathers, and had been tomboys as young girls. In the late 1960s, maybe these women were trying to express to the psychiatrists some latent feelings about women's roles that had not even emerged yet under the banner of women's liberation.

Two types of mother personalities were pinned down as models to be rejected: either the controlling, rejecting mother or, by contrast, the passive, downtrodden mother.

From that point on, deciding that I would not be able to rely solely on these psychoanalytic opinions, I returned to my own form of research and added a question to those interviews I felt were deep enough—I asked the women about their relationship with their mothers. Half expecting them to say it was none of my business, or that their mother was the dearest person to their hearts, I was often surprised to hear every woman I asked express her own deep feelings about the rejection of this significant woman in her life.

We would comment on our shared vehemence, and tried to examine together why this should be. The answers were not easy to find, nor were they altogether welcome. Jeanne N., a thirty-five-year-old book editor, for example, whose own mother had worked all her young life, leaving Jeanne to be brought up by nannies, would appear to have had a very different background from my own (my mother was a traditional housewife).

OUR MOTHERS' EXPERIENCE OF PPD

We must not forget that our mothers may also have gone through PPD and, not knowing what it was, probably refused to admit to it. Denial is a common reaction even today. In past generations, however, it must have been hard, if not impossible, to reject the mothering role, the only one freely given to women; to say they had found unhappiness in motherhood, when nothing else was permitted them.

I received several retrospective comments from women, such as this: "I will never forget that dreadful year after my son was born, and that was twenty-one years ago. It was the loneliest time of my life, and I did not know it was PPD, or that it was anything that had a name."

Confronted by her daughter's PPD, Nancy E.'s mother at first snapped, "Get on with dealing with your two children and pull yourself together." But she did open up after the psychiatrist lent the family a pamphlet on depression. Nancy now believes her mother experienced a heavy PPD, too, but still has not really owned up to it.

"When my sister was born, my mother nearly died from toxemia. That was her second child in three years. For a year afterward, she never saw a doctor, or talked about it to anyone, but she feared she was losing her mind. She was very depressed, had anxiety attacks, and would be sitting talking to friends wondering if they could see she was going insane. She had three children in six years, never worked, never got out of the house much, and never complained. I think that's why I really used to believe women were supposed to be utterly self-sacrificing when they were mothers."

When Kathy S. tried to be honest about her feelings with her mother, she was told sharply, "Why have a child if you feel like that?" Kathy's mother continued to reject her daughter, as she had all her life. When I asked Kathy directly about this relationship with her mother, she said sadly, "We never got on, we were never close. One of my first reactions to having my baby, because of the image I carried still of her—always unhappy, tied down, complaining—was, 'Oh no, I'm going to be old and stuck like my mother.' I didn't even want Joe to call me mommy. I hated the sound of the word!

"From the time I was seven," explained Kathy, "until I was nineteen and left home to get married, I knew my mother was unhappy. She told me her problems and made me feel I had to look after her.

"To this day I'm the dominant woman in the family, the one who holds it all together. My mother lives on the same street, won't drive a car, is dependent on me and still critical. I had been married six years to Bill before getting pregnant. Somehow I hoped it might bring me and my mother closer together. She is a strict Catholic, and from the age of twelve she had warned me not to get pregnant out of marriage or she would throw me out of the house. Here I was at twenty-five, married six years, coming to tell her I was pregnant, and I was shivering with nervousness in case she was angry. She wasn't exactly thrilled or elated, but passed it off without much comment."

Kathy grew up with an image of her mother as a downtrodden, passive woman. "If only she'd had some money of her own, she might have been happier, I knew that even as a child." It should have been no surprise to Kathy, therefore, that she was determined to go back to work after having her baby, that she openly expressed fear of staying home all the time with her child. Yet the conflicts within herself clouded that reality. Kathy wanted to be a real mother; but in her mind being a real mother meant being unhappy.

If a woman's mother was cold or rejecting, when she has her own baby, she wants to give that child all the love she was denied. For Sharon W., with two daughters under four, the rejection by her mother was specific and awful. Her stepfather had sexually abused her over several years. Sharon's mother never knew about it, or pretended not to know. "She never had time for me. My sister was born ten months later, and there were three of us before she was twenty-one. I was raised by my grandparents much of the time." In therapy, Sharon began to learn something of herself and her behavior with her own daughters. "I started to see I was trying to break my elder daughter's spirit, just like my mother had broken mine." In an effort to draw closer to her mother after all these years, Sharon tried to explain over the telephone just what had gone on with her stepfather. But confronting her mother with the truth left Sharon feeling even more rejected, for her mother refused to believe the story.

Women have unfortunately been guilty of furthering PPD through the generations in this desire to cover up or deny their real feelings after childbirth. By staying silent, handing on the burden to their daughters with comments like "This is how life is, so just grow up and get on with it," they have helped perpetuate various myths rather than deal with the reality, which might alleviate much of the guilt and shame for what are genuine, acceptable, feelings.

Maybe if we are able to be open, less guilty, more comfortable with the ambivalence and negative feelings, we will begin to improve the situation for our daughters. Just as we intend to be open about menstruation and about sex and female sexuality, to discuss our own emotions and theirs in human, loving, honest ways, maybe we should prepare ourselves to discuss with our sons and daughters our response to motherhood, not in a negative way, but with honesty.

I believe some of our sadness after birth is part of a greater genetic endowment; that we carry within us the misery of women in the past, some of the despair of being trapped that our mothers and grandmothers might have experienced. Culturally, we associate becoming a mother with turning from independent, autonomous people—a victory so recently won—to passive, oppressed, overextended, and underappreciated less-than-human beings.

Even though up to conception, and during pregnancy, we were inspired with the greatest optimism that *we would be doing it differently,* once that baby was in our arms, we suddenly understood and appreciated our forebears more vividly than ever before: we suddenly identified *too* fully with them. Many women have said that only on becoming a mother did they feel real sympathy with their own mothers. As one of my correspondents put it, "A mother's guilt is something that binds all mothers together."

MOTHER LONGING

Therese Benedek takes us to a deeper analytical root of PPD. When we give birth, we regress to the oral phase, which, she says, is the main psychogenic condition for depression, involving the "female child's identification with its mother."[46]

When we give birth, all our own infantile instincts and reactions are reactivated. For some women that might mean reliving ambivalence about our mothers that we experienced as infants: the desire to be separate and the need to merge with her. When we hear our own baby crying, it might stimulate our own feelings of being newborn, our desire to be loved and nourished. Most of us feel a strong urge to be mothered during pregnancy and just after the birth, which is symbolic of the confusion deep within us.

In a long article about the reconstruction of the life of a woman suffering a difficult PPD, psychoanalyst Harold Blum concluded, "How could she be the mother of a separate, living, unique individual when she *wanted* and *dreaded* to be fused with her mother, clinging and separating, regressively eating rather than feeding and caring for her own infant?"[47]

Thirty-year-old Dianne McL. experienced just this type of reactivation when crying heavily in the first few days after her baby's birth. "I stumbled on the reason for it myself. Although I had been in therapy for years, I had never touched on this. I was reexperiencing the pain of separation from my real mother, and this was why I had wanted a child so much, to experience that sense of bonding I had missed out on."

Dianne openly admitted to being a recovering alcoholic who had also had drug problems, and a member of Alcoholics Anonymous for three years (the last two of which she had been sober). The alcohol problem was connected with this oral longing for her mother's love, and yet, after years of intensive psychotherapy and AA, she had not touched on this very real need in her.

Dianne and her brother had been adopted by their aunt and her husband when Dianne was eighteen months old. Their mother, deemed unfit to care for them, was admitted to a mental institution shortly afterward. Tragically for Dianne's mother, no one was much concerned about the cause of her mental problem and, as Dianne put it, "If she was not insane when she went in there, she certainly would be by now, twenty-five years later."[48]

Dianne had said something very important, and it resonated in me. She was crying for the pain of separation from her own mother. She was crying for the ambivalence, for the love she never received enough of, for the bonding she yearned for and missed. She was crying for her mother's sad fate, with which she was now forced to identify. For most of her young adult life Dianne had not given much thought to the woman in the asylum, knowing only her adoptive mother and devoting more energy to thinking about that dynamic and often difficult relationship.

Mother and daughter is a complex relationship, and our responses cannot be passed off glibly as "problems with the feminine role" or "a mothering conflict."

SECOND OR THIRD CHILD

A fascinating aspect of rejecting our mothers comes in the explanation of why we may not suffer PPD with a first baby, but with a second or third child. If our mother had more than one child, we may have successfully avoided identifying ourselves in her image until we suddenly found ourselves with the *same number* of children. Judith Klein explains further:

"The female child, in the Oedipal stage, had to turn from loving her mother to having strong sexual feelings for the parent of the opposite sex. In rejecting her mother, and desiring ultimately to have sex with her father, and bear *his* child, she invoked the image of her mother's retaliation and anger, which led to the child's own anxiety and guilt. Oedipal problems may be compounded and not resolved if the child's father was especially close to her and, to some degree, seductive. I am not even referring to sexual abuse or incest, but to a handsome, adoring daddy who seduces his own daughter into continuing her Oedipal desire for him beyond the normal stage.

"One way a young adult woman may react, to keep such fear and anxieties at bay, is in avoiding having a baby, or avoiding getting married. If married she may deliberately have affairs, try to destroy the marriage, or refuse to play the traditional female role. Another way of avoidance is to have *one less child* than her mother did. While she has one less she is conscious of being different and of not being in direct competition with her."

PPD after the birth of a second, or third, child may be the result of reactivated unresolved Oedipal conflicts, early anxiety, depression, or guilt, a sense of competition with the mother, or perhaps contempt for her ("Daddy prefers me to you"), and, concurrently, fear of identifying with the mother's apparent "female" role.

This brings me back to the generational theory. If a woman today has, to one degree or another, rejected her mother's lifestyle; felt contempt for her version of housewife-mother; felt pity for her lack of independence, money of her own, or ability to act a part in the greater world; or felt pity for her lack of sexual power and freedom, is this woman then more likely to suffer from the psychological causes of PPD? I cannot answer that. But we are living through transitional times and it is unlikely that we will all sail through unscathed.

THE "WELL-ADJUSTED" WOMAN

There is a popular image that a well-adjusted woman does not suffer from PPD; that certain personality types are more likely to make a good mother and adjust better to mothering. Other types, in the same vision, are on a disaster course even before they have conceived.

Women likely to get PPD are variously seen as those who are narcissistic, obsessional, compliant, conformist, oversensitive, have a controlling personality, are defensive against the primitive in life, married to a passive/dominant husband, or in a marriage where both husband and wife are mutually dependent. Certain traits are seen as proof that the woman had a defective personality before becoming a mother: the fault cannot possibly lie with motherhood so it *must* lie with these foolish women.

Such PPD mothers would have predisposing neurotic tendencies; for example, as a child, they would have displayed nail biting, excessive fear of the dark, shyness, night terrors, sleep walking, temper tantrums, stammering.[49]

PPD women are commonly viewed as being overdependent on their husbands or seeking a mother in their spouses. It has even been suggested that a woman whose husband does housework has a defective personality, presumably because she allows him to do such female work![50] However, these theories were propounded twenty or thirty years ago, and who would have guessed men would turn in droves to doing the housework! Psychiatrist Gregory Zilboorg wrote in 1957 that women who reject their children by spending all day at their own pursuits, hiring a nanny or governess to care for the children, show a basic hostility toward mothering and are classic candidates for PPD.[51] Maybe we cannot expect to learn too much about ourselves from such psychoanalytic pronouncements.

I doubt there is a personality type that predisposes any of us to PPD. We all undergo the same hormonal changes. For some of us, intensive external pressures, whether from responsibilities, relationship and role fluctuations, loss of identity, or confusion over ourselves as women and now mothers, will place undue burden on the hypothalamic-pituitary network, leading to a crisis among the neurohormones—and consequent symptoms of PPD. The cheerful, idealistic, optimistic woman who sees herself as the strong member of the family is just as likely to experience PPD as is the neurotic, sad type of woman.

"I'm not a schizophrenic, I'm strong," cried Kathy S. on first learning of that diagnosis of her PPD symptoms. But now, with much greater understanding and awareness, she can admit and accept its roots and causes in her own life. "Out of my entire life, having my son has been the most significant and shattering event. It wasn't getting married, or going back to college, that affected me so totally. But just becoming a mother."

Laura S. commented, "When you are in a successful career the idea of depression seems ridiculous. I was used to knowing what I wanted to do, going for it, and succeeding. But dealing with my child was something so unpredictable, I couldn't put him or motherhood in any category, it was not like anything I'd read or done before."

Becoming a parent may shock and surprise us when it brings back angry childhood feelings to people or relationships. Conflicts with mother or father, siblings, or authority figures, depressions from the past, fear of separation or by being submerged, fear of being trapped, may all float dangerously near the surface after long being buried.

For myself, being a parent, not so much of babies but of young preschoolers, brought back depressive feelings I had experienced as a child and adolescent: of entrapment, boredom, a fear that I would never get anywhere or do anything significant in my life. Old anger at my parents' control over me became a repressed anger at the control my children were now exerting over me and my life.

When I was newly and so proudly pregnant for the first time, I remember going to see an editor who had given me a break with my first book. Feeling flushed with my triumph, for the book was to be published in the same year my baby would be born (it felt like a double birth), expecting the usual congratulatory platitudes with which we greet pregnant women socially, I was floored by the rather dour comment, "What on earth do you want a baby for? What's wrong with your life now?" He was a father himself, so I could not put his comment down totally to that male selfishness of not wanting children to clutter up their lives.

I laughed off the question at the time, yet it has stayed with me, lingering to be reawakened while I was writing this book. What an interesting question it was. I like the second part best. "What's wrong with your life now?" I can recall thinking petulantly, "Nothing, of course. This baby will be an extension of my life with my husband, not a narrowing." The idealism, the romantic fantasies, that fuel our drive to reproduce; that image of ourselves as mothers and fathers. But his question had a point. A baby will change the life we have now, whether we accept or deny that change. We should be aware of and prepared for the change. We do not really have to come up with good reasons for wanting babies other than a deep desire, or love for our partners, or wish to perpetuate the species. We will be forced, however, by subconscious or conscious pressures to think out our new lives, alter habits, relearn new life patterns, new psychological survival instincts, before we can move on as parents. PPD is a time of mourning; for saying goodbye to childless freedom and identity. Hello to . . . we are not quite sure what.

PART THREE

Working Mothers

Chapter 10

DEALING WITH THE CHOICES

When we consider mothers who work either full time or part time out of the home or are self-employed in the home, and when we consider mothers who have given up work to be home full time with their children, we are tackling one enormously complex subject of image, identity, role expectations, and personal energy levels. In this section of the book we will look in depth at these problems and concerns. Time and again women asked me to treat the problems of working mothers seriously; nor would I want to underestimate the position of the nonworking mothers. Both come to their motherhood with hopes, desires, fantasies, and an expectation that their chosen path will lead to happiness. No less than those issues brought up in the last section, the whole topic of work or not to work leads women to the particular stresses and strains of PPD. The "why do I feel like this when I should be so happy?" question is a common complaint of women led to believe they have been offered choices, have accepted the offer, and expect roses all the way.

Just as with any other form of stress or psychological confusion, the biochemical disruption can be extensive for a new mother dealing not only with becoming a mother but with that very real bewildering muddle of just what her image is, as woman, worker, and a mother.

Think of the dreams we harbored as small girls, teenagers, and young women, of what we would be like as mothers. No doubt most of us fondly imagined giving up work—if work was in our fantasies at all—to stay home and be perfect mothers. Think of the expectations fostered by our own mothers, husbands, mothers-in-law, friends, and colleagues, that no real mother ever works. Pit those images against our own complex self-assessment. On the one hand, we know we have an interesting job, perhaps even a passionate commitment to a career, we enjoy the companionship of working, and we appreciate the financial independence and the extra income for the family. On the other hand, we are not sure if those are valid justifications for continuing to work after the baby is born. We fear society's condemnation of us as self-indulgent, as cold, rejecting mothers; we fear our inadequacy as women and failure as mothers.

Take that particular psychological stew, add to it complications from unavailable, expensive, frightening, or unknown childcare options, criticism from relatives, colleagues, and friends, and you have a deep pot of potential trouble that can all too easily lead to PPD.

This is a very gender-oriented concern. Few men ever face the question of whether becoming a parent may mean the loss of their work life. How do women make their choice? Unfortunately for most of us, the road to decision is haphazard, wavering, and often arrived at by default. One reason for the sometimes chronic indecisiveness is that we underestimate ourselves.

We are not just *one* person, straight as a die, sticking resolutely to one set of beliefs and ideas. When Freud asked, "What do women really want?" no one could give an answer. We are all mixtures of possibilities, limitations, genetic predisposition, and environmental supports and pressures. I know one part of me sees an intellectual bohemian, a Vita Sackville-West type, who should have been born to greater wealth and status to indulge in writing and the grand life, leaving others to deal with the domestic, mundane, daily maternal duties. Another side of me longs to be a mother like my own mother: devoted, caring, concerned, involved, always there, seemingly content to lead that proscribed life of husband, home, and children. Yet another side would like to live somewhere exotic, with a husband who did not have to work all day, surrounded by a brood of children, devoting my life to a social, carefree existence, forgetting all worldly pursuits.

Just because we have become mothers does not mean that we all have the same needs and desires. Some of us suffer guilt from returning to work because secretly we prefer to *work* than to mother. Some of us resent working because secretly we would prefer to be *mothering.* Others are just plain confused and conflicted, unable to put a finger on what we would rather be doing, on what would make us happiest. Some of us resent that we need to work for money, and deep down feel that our husbands should be able to provide. Some of us resent the implication that we are selfish because we want to work. These confusions over what we think we should, or would really like to, be doing are easy stimuli of PPD.

GOING BACK TO WORK, NOT REALLY WANTING TO

We cannot guess during pregnancy how we will feel once the baby is born. While pregnant, many of us make conscious decisions that we will have our babies and continue to work, knowing full well we enjoy our jobs, need the money, and are convinced we would not be happy staying home as a housewife. Yet, when the real baby is in our arms, a different vision shades our eyes.

Some find it very hard to leave a new baby in those early weeks, even with a husband, mother, or trusted baby-sitter. The thought of going back to work begins to prey on our minds, growing out of all proportion as an enormous threat. We panic. We are consumed by guilt and anxiety, and depression sets in.

Two women, at different ends of the career spectrum, found out just how unexpected these maternal feelings can be. Gina C. was a twenty-five-year-old analyst for an insurance firm in her hometown, and had been married only a year when her son was born. She had always planned to go back to work. As her firm promised to hold the job open for six weeks, she had to commit herself to that small amount of time off. Gina feared that a lengthier leave of absence might jeopardize her job.

But tiredness and the strangeness of becoming a mother, compounded by worries about money, possible loss of the job, and leaving the baby, left her so badly depressed and given to uncontrollable crying spells that she was in no fit state to return to work once the six weeks were up.

Gina had become phobic about leaving her child, even with her own mother. She never went out with her husband, and their relationship slid quickly into decline. "I couldn't understand the way I was feeling. I was aggressively hostile toward my husband, as well as suffering the depression. I just knew I was an awful person who had wanted for years to settle down and have children. Now all I could do was cry and act hateful."

In the end, Gina extended her leave of absence to two and a half months. Finally the day came when she had to return to the office, desperate with fear, anxiety, and guilt. Her depression was such that "it felt like a conspiracy to keep my child away from me. I resented everyone at work as if it were their fault."

Gina's resentment was a symptom of severe PPD. Knowing nothing about it, she struggled on with work and her conflicting emotions. To make matters worse, she had a new boss who seemed to hate women in general. "His view was that women were just a burden to the work force. If they weren't having babies they were having hysterectomies, and he would do everything he could to get rid of them. I'm sure he thought I'd quit when he put me in a new position I hated."

Still burdened by an uncontrollable desire to cry, Gina would hide in the bathroom, to avoid seeming weak. Slowly her personality returned to normal as she reconciled being a mother and being out of the house all day, and her hormonal system had time to settle down along with her psyche.

Marsha H. had planned to return to her work because, as a television producer, she had struggled to gain her position for years. The birth of a first child, at age thirty-five, did not seem reason enough to give it all up. The money she and Bob were bringing in afforded them a comfortable lifestyle with household help, to which both were adjusted and loath to lose.

Once Jason was born, however, the self-assured Marsha was no longer certain that she even liked her work or wanted to stay on. "Work is no simple solution for women. I went back full time at first, but had to take a downward drop in position, and a salary cut, just to be able to cope. I used to think about Jason all the time. He was constantly on my mind. I was useless at work." She finally opted to work a four-day week on three-quarters salary, and said ironically, "Then I was busy trying to get into a *more* boring job than that, so I could work just a six-day fortnight."

Marsha moved down from producer's level to what she called a hack job, something she could do with only half her mind. She was fortunate to be able to make such a decision. But Marsha was already afflicted with a very strong case of PPD before she even returned to work. She opted contentedly for the compromise of a less significant position at work, on lower pay, which allowed her more time at home with her baby. Marsha had discovered she did not want the full-time professional career if it prevented her from mothering effectively.

The experience of PPD for many women does seem to offer a time for reassessment of values and priorities in life. The crisis brought about by uncontrollable emotions and psychological warfare forces theories and judgments into the open—even if they are only argued about at least they are voiced.

GIVING UP WORK, NOT REALLY HAPPY

"I was used to feeling busy, useful, and independent, then all of a sudden everything changed," wrote Pamela B. about her experience after the birth of her first child. At age thirty-two, with a job in an advertising agency, she left work, giving no commitment on when she would return, imagining she would love being home with her baby. By the fifth month, Pamela knew she had to get back to work or she would go out of her mind. Being at home with her child was not the dream she had imagined.

Pamela was perhaps typical of a lot of women today. Go-getting, not necessarily aggressive or ambitious at work, but determined to have a good, full, and interesting life, before becoming a mother she had held down a full-time job, worked out at the gym, practiced karate, enjoyed aerobics, took music lessons, traveled, got enough sleep, and even had time for her husband and to socialize. Pamela kept up the busy pace to the day of delivery.

"And then what?" she exclaimed. Suffering PPD for four months, she felt dragged out and lethargic, trapped by the daily routine of caring for a baby. She had lost blood until the ninth week postpartum, which accentuated her feeling of fatigue. She resented her husband's freedom and was anxious about money. "All through the pregnancy, I was well supported and looked forward to being a mother. But this felt like being put out to pasture to fend for myself alone at a very crucial time."

For Pamela, PPD had come on about a month after the baby's birth, when she had time and energy enough to realize that her whole previous way of life had changed and that the fantasized image of herself at home with her baby was not coming true. Pamela ran the gamut of typical PPD emotions. "That dragged out, lethargic, trapped" feeling was earlier described as the later-onset type of PPD (compared to the anxious, agitated, often hallucinatory type of PPD that begins in the first week or two after birth).

Pamela's case was not bad enough to send her to a doctor. But she did return to work, and she forced herself back into a routine of exercise. Slowly, her hormonal system returned to normal, and she began to feel more like her old self.

EAGER TO RETURN TO WORK

Kathy S. accepted early on that she was happiest back at work. "I was *glad* to be back there. I couldn't wait to get away from the house," she said. Kathy knew that being at home all day would make her feel trapped, financially dependent, and unhappy—as her mother had been. She adjusted to her role of working mother more easily than to her role of mother. Yet she came in for plenty of social criticism. Other women at work made sure Kathy heard their comments: "Your child is suffering and you don't need the second paycheck." But Kathy had inner strength from the conviction that being at home with her child would *not* be the best possible solution for either of them.

As we have seen earlier from Kathy's story, the eagerness to get back to work and out of the house was her open admission that full-time motherhood was too hard for her to handle. Kathy had woken up from her c-section delivery wishing she could walk out of the hospital alone. She had not wanted to be associated with her mother. She had not wanted her son to call her mommy. How could the PPD have come upon her so quickly? As far as medical opinion is concerned, PPD symptoms cannot show themselves before the third day postpartum, when the initial hormonal shifts have taken place and sown the seeds for distress. In Kathy's case, the psychological confusion was there in her mind from the minute she gave birth. Her mind had begun working in this negative and distressing way even before the hormonal upheaval. Kathy has described herself as nonfunctional as a mother for at least six months from the time she and her husband took Joe home. Eventually, although they never sought any outside help, as the baby developed happily, as she picked up her working life and outside interests, Kathy's body resettled and she was emotionally able to accept Joe as her son, and herself as his mother.

FLOUNDERING IN INDECISION

Other women flounder in confusion. Aileen B. was just such a case. She was twenty-five when she had her daughter, and had worked until that time as a teacher. Aileen and her husband, John, were not planning a family, for she had had an ovary removed and had been told a number of times that she could never conceive. Baby Jennifer's birth was therefore an utter delight. As the couple had a huge mortgage to feed, Aileen returned to teaching soon after the birth. Aileen described going into such a period of gloom after her return to work that it was the most difficult and disturbing time of her life, because being a working mother went against her deepest wishes and dreams.

"The rest of the world believed it was my responsibility to stay home with the baby and I tended to agree. Finally I gave in to popular demand and compromised by getting a part-time job, doing some teaching in the evenings. My husband worked days and we felt it would be the best of all worlds as we would be with the baby twenty-four hours a day." But then things grew worse. For one thing, they had very little money, and this made Aileen feel trapped. She and her husband had no time together; all their time was for the baby. Aileen felt totally inadequate dealing with Jennifer, and that sense of inadequacy was made worse by everyone telling her to pull herself together and get on with being a wife and mother.

"The depression finally ended when I took control of the situation and went back to work full time," she said. Their marriage survived the stress and, with her return to work for a few years, they managed to clear up some of their financial mess. Then Aileen left work again. "I felt motherhood was my real job, and the one I was happiest with," she commented on her final decision.

Confusion, conflict, weighing the pros and cons . . . one twenty-seven-year-old mother who felt she was forced back to work realized two or three months later that she was really feeling tremendous relief, and consequent guilt, at not being home with her baby. When she confessed to a colleague one day, "It feels good to be back at work," the friend replied wryly, "You mean you almost feel bad about feeling good."

PPD, in these cases of chronic confusion, will only lift when somehow the mother is able to confront the conflicting forces battling it out within her and make a compromise that is right for *her*, not for society.

COMPROMISES

Many working women have found compromises in three- or four-day weeks, or perhaps have arranged to finish their day by 4 P.M. so the child is not in alternative care all day. The choice means putting their career on hold, but, ideally, positions will be there when they resume at full speed a few years later, or the compromise will have shown them that their part-time status suits them.

Even a shortened working week will not magically overcome all the exhaustion and confusion of the dual-role conflict. Married to a successful international businessman, Jeanne N., the thirty-five-year-old book editor, had achieved a certain status in her career before she had her two children. Because she had a live-in baby-sitter who stayed with the family three days and nights a week (and alternate weekends), anyone might assume that she was privileged enough to make an easy and successful blend of career and motherhood. Jeanne did not really want to put her career on hold, but she did want to be able to spend time with her children, so she arranged to work a three-day week in the office and be paid for a four-day week, making up the time at home. Surely someone like Jeanne would not suffer PPD.

The situation has worked out fine for her company, but maybe not so fine for Jeanne. Admittedly compulsive about her work, every evening she would rush out of the office to be home by six-thirty. She had her children in bed by seven-thirty or eight, and then would continue her office work. "My husband traveled a lot and worked late hours too, so it was possible to be still working till ten or eleven—but it was exhausting!" she said.

"I really should have had full-time help. I don't believe now you can do part-time work with part-time help. How can you edit an author's book, or talk with another publisher, when you have a screaming toddler and a four-year-old boy who hates to see you work? I had worked the housekeeping arrangement out that she was there when I was not. That meant the days I was not in the office, I also had to spend time with, or take care of, the children.

"My own mother was amazed I chose this option, because I had hated that she worked when I was a child. Once when she asked me what I wanted for Christmas, I had said, 'A mommy who stays home'! My son does the same to me. He sounds like an orphan sometimes. He'll catch me dressing for work in the morning and wail, 'Who's going to take care of me today?' Then, when I do stay home, he's so excited it's very touching. It isn't easy, is it?"

Jeanne was talking about the experience of trying to be good at both—profession and mothering—with a sinking feeling that she had failed at both. "You want to present a competent image—say to an author—of a working woman and a mother. Then, when they call you, your child is screaming and you feel like a bad mother for not heeding her, or, like a lousy professional for saying to the author, 'I'm sorry I can't do this now, my son hasn't seen me all day.' "

Jeanne was also talking about the kind of PPD that becomes a permanent fixture in our lives: born of the fatigue women obviously feel juggling two or more roles, it is fed by anxiety, tension, the stresses of keeping up with different lives, with pleasing different people—and very often, that ultimate stress of having nothing left over for you.

Jeanne, the woman who had everything, also had an underlying, constant, nagging level of PPD—things were just not quite right.

THE TRIPLE WHAMMY

Women in clerical positions, secretaries, nurses, teachers, or those in the service industries may find their bosses very unsympathetic to the needs or concerns of new mothers. It may not be possible for them to work flex-time hours, or a three- to four-day week, or to finish early in the afternoon. The employer may begin from a position of suspicion that the new mother will be exploiting him or her in taking sick days to look after her child. These women may also find themselves returning to work earlier than women with more flexible jobs, fearing loss of pay, loss of their job, or criticism from within the workplace.

All working mothers are vulnerable to the triple whammy: being pulled apart by loyalties to baby, husband, and job; feeling guilt at not giving any of the triad enough of their time and energy; being exhausted from trying. Ideally, no working woman should have to return to work until at least three months after a baby is born, and preferably nearer five months. By the fifth month the baby should be sleeping longer at night, freeing the mother to cope with a working day. Also, the five-month-old infant will be beginning to show signs of independence, so that leaving him or her is not as wrenching an experience for either mother or child.

If coming home from work proves to be little joy for the harried new mother: if it means struggling to prepare an evening meal, make up bottles, put the baby down, clean the house, and shortly thereafter fall asleep herself, depression may not be far behind. Julia F. was seriously depressed when, after returning to her customer service job eight weeks after the c-section delivery of her baby, total exhaustion had almost literally drained the life out of her. Her doctor suggested antidepressant medication but was unsympathetic to her condition and would not sign a statement for sick leave. Julia described the feeling of the triple whammy: "There just wasn't enough of me to go around."

Fatigue that is experienced by any woman after giving birth will be felt acutely by a mother who has returned to work and who tries to cram too much into one short day.

RESPECTING FATIGUE AS A WARNING SIGNAL

Exhaustion, fatigue, call it what you will, must be the single most common warning of potential collapse of the hormonal system. Trying to do everything, assuming we can handle all our new roles at once, can lead us down the fast track to total disintegration. Dr. Elisabeth Herz put it this way: "Modern women think they can have it all, and I don't blame them. They want both career and motherhood, and why not? But they fail to understand that they must compromise somewhere along the line. They may try everything—but they cannot do it all to perfection."

When the feelings of fatigue and being overstretched just won't go away, something has to give. It may be the hours put in at work, the amount of domestic work done after work hours, the time we can give the baby and other children, or time for our husband. If something doesn't give, the giving-out will come from the new mother.

Liz H. was thirty-three and the mother of a third child, just six weeks old, when she returned to work as an administrative assistant at a local college. Not having worked during the other two children's young years, she was eager to be back with adult company and away from the house.

With classes beginning, work was very heavy in those early weeks of fall, and Liz put in ten- to twelve-hour days, six days a week, for a whole month. "I was so mentally and physically exhausted that at home I screamed at my elder daughters and was unresponsive to my husband. I did not know what was happening to me. But I knew I was on the verge of cracking up. I seriously considered suicide, which is why, looking back, the whole thing was so frightening. I didn't even know I was depressed until my doctor referred me to a psychiatrist, who suggested it. I hadn't seen any of the warning signals because I'd never suffered a severe depression before.

"All I know is I didn't care about anything. I cried frequently and was absolutely miserable. I just thought I was a terrible person. I really wish more was known about PPD. It would make it so much easier if we felt we were not the only ones going through this. The joke is I went back to my obstetrician to tell him about it, and to say it seems I had PPD. He didn't agree with me!"

Liz had never been depressed before, she knew nothing about PPD, and she failed to connect her warning signals. Liz had never given her system time to settle down with the heavy responsibilities found at work. More than that, because she had stayed home when her other daughters were babies, she no doubt felt confused about her new role as working mother. The overload on her body and mind was evident.

QUALITY TIME OR QUANTITY TIME?

"Quality time" has become the watchword from the battle lines of the beleaguered working mother camp. Indeed, the plethora of playgroups, nursery schools, and day camp activities that are available in most cities and many towns for children whose mothers do *not* go to work is evidence that society has caught up. Many mothers now accept that a young child may be happier *not* spending all his or her time with the mother alone. Even experts like Dr. Spock have grudgingly admitted that it is good for mothers to have time to themselves, for babies and toddlers to learn to mix with others, to play in groups.[52]

As Dr. Herz comments, however, "quality time" should not be used by working mothers to justify too little time with their children. A young child does need a lot of both the mother's and father's time, since some *quantity* of time is necessary to make it quality time. All our interactions with our children need not be happy, cuddly, or adventurous. There is space in our lives for argument, irritation, and boredom as well. A child who grows up feeling comfortable with these emotions from his or her own parents will find dealing with the outside world less bewildering.

A very busy working mother, with a full-time career that demands long hours away from home, with maybe a commute there and back adding to those hours, and additional "homework" hours, may find herself with little time on a *daily* basis with her baby or young child and can suffer consequent acute guilt that she may be depriving her child of some fundamental nurturing care that should be offered by the mother. And she may be right.

What if you cannot see your child every morning and every evening, at least; or what if whole days go by without him or her catching sight of you in your smart work clothes or even nightclothes? Guilt is one of the strongest emotions felt by new mothers. Forget love, happiness, or warm nurturing feelings, most women probably know guilt better than they do love! Very often the mother who has such a hectic schedule has already come to a compromise with her husband that he will be able to take some of the childcare shifts. Maybe she has a close relative who is able to be around the home for stretches at a time: certainly the constant love of a grandparent is highly beneficial to a young child.

Before any of us looks accusingly at a new mother, we should bear in mind that for generations, wealthy families in Britain and Europe, and many in the United States, hired outsiders—nannies, governesses, au pairs—and that the mothers and fathers were conspicuously absent in the day-to-day raising of the children. For centuries, even further back in history, women of high birth used wet nurses to breastfeed their children, and those new mothers probably had little contact with their children until they were at least on their feet and able to mouth polite endearments to their mothers.

It is only very recently, in the twentieth century, that society or women themselves have deemed it necessary for the mother to be with her child at all times—up to whatever age the expert of the moment says it is healthy for her to do so—or maintained that only the mother can offer good nurturing care for her child. I cannot accept that all those children from past centuries grew up emotionally deprived if their mothers did not personally devote their undivided attention to their infancy.

In a recent article on the subject, called "The Working Mother as Role Model," Anita Shreve reported that experts had found many positive side effects to the current increase in mothers working out of the house for long hours of the day. Dr. Samuel Ritvo and Dr. Kyle Pruett, professors of psychiatry at Yale University, presented evidence that seeing mother and father as nurturer and achiever had been good for children of either sex. Shreve wrote, "Child specialists suggest that the next generation of women may be less troubled about pursuing both 'masculine' and 'feminine' endeavors. Women may be able more easily to combine career and family life—a juggling act that stymies many women today and often leads to feelings of inadequacy, stress and guilt."[53]

Shreve quotes Betty Friedan as saying, "The daughters of women today are more assertive and have a clearer sense of themselves. They will have both their careers and their children without guilt." Boys too are seen to gain from having working mothers, as they may grow into men more sensitive to the needs of women. "The next generation of lawmakers, both men and women, will have had mothers who are working women," said Friedan.

I know from the women I have met that busy professional working mothers, or those working awkward shifts, go to great lengths to give time to their children—often to the detriment of their personal lives.

Having a child does mean taking time out of our own lives. A child does feed off some part of us, devours some portion of our former selves. No relationship can grow without long stretches of time together. Relations between husband and wife wither and die if they spend too much time apart. But children can feel mothering tangibly in her care and concern, in a warm, happy, secure, interesting home—not only in her daily physical presence and ability to bake cookies.

Of course there have always been parents who have been negligent of their children, in their absence or in the lack of love or life in their homes. One new mother, Mary S., was very much aware of that kind of negligence while, ironically, ensnaring herself in a way of life that very nearly carried on the sins of her parents to her own child.

Mary: On the Treadmill

Newspaper reporter Mary S. had in some ways condemned herself to exhaustion, because the housekeeper who took care of fifteen-month-old Noah was employed to be there only when Mary or her husband, Bruce, were out of the apartment. This meant that Mary had no time to herself. There was not a minute of the day, she explained, that was not preordained to some duty. The minute Mary or Bruce returned home, the housekeeper left for the day. Mary had no time for creative projects, for putting away her winter clothes, or for paying bills. In the end, even Mary saw she had to devise a different plan for all their sakes. One of her new resources was to take *more* time from her daily newspaper job to be with Noah. Somehow by giving him more time, she felt less that she was being robbed of her own. So, instead of lunch one day she took Noah to a birthday party. One morning a week, she arranged to go in to work later so she could take him, herself, to a neighborhood playgroup with other mothers.

Mary was perhaps made aware of the dangers of not being with a child for enough time, from her own childhood experience. Her mother had never worked, yet she and her brother were brought up by housekeepers (her father died when she was two). "I don't even remember going on vacation with my mother, and my brother and I had a very unhappy childhood. I was always separated from my parents, which is probably why I have found leaving Noah so traumatic.

"I have tried to give him a stable routine. I don't leave for work until nearly eleven, and one of us is home by six-thirty or seven-thirty. We spend time with Noah and he goes to bed quite happily before eight. He really seems content, which is why I hope we are doing something right."

We met Mary previously in the section on older mothers. Having just turned forty, juggling to keep up a working life on the newspaper, her personal creative life as a writer of art history books, some semblance of a social life with her husband (and a professional social life too), and be a mother to Noah, she confessed then that she felt so wracked by a mental rather than physical exhaustion that she had become very absentminded and anxiety-ridden. She was perpetually rushing to be places, get projects finished, with a sense of always failing. Mary was suffering a mild version of PPD that emerges as a chronic condition—it may go on throughout the child's early life and continue through the birth of the next baby. The fatigue, confusion, juggling of roles, guilt induced by her own mother's negligence, and fears that she herself would not be a good mother to Noah, had all contrived to create this state of just-barely-ticking-by exhaustion so common in many working mothers today.

CHILDCARE WITHOUT GUILT

Childcare that helps the mother as much as it helps the child may be the most important investment we make in our working-mother lives. Childcare is big business. More than 62 percent of families (in the United States) have both parents out in the workplace (an increase from 40 percent in 1960). In a survey of 5 million mothers with at least one child of preschool age, taken in June 1982, 14.8 percent placed their child in a nursery school or day care center, and 22 percent left their child for some part of the day in the home of a nonrelative.

Despite occasional scares about the safety and reliability of day care centers, or the qualifications of nursery schools, the vast majority operate responsibly. There is as yet in the United States no government protection of these private institutions, and even little checking in the states on how they are run. It is left to the parents to judge the institution, whether the fees are appropriate, whether the childcare is good, and whether they are happy with the care givers.

The flare-ups that reach our eyes about badly run or abusive centers always give ammunition to the anti-working-mother brigade. But, if we can assume that women work for reasonable and realistic choices, that children would not necessarily be any happier if we all stayed home full time, after we have checked out the particular institution we should look at how the form of childcare is working for *us*. Stressful childcare arrangements will aggravate PPD.

For a newborn's care, the ideal situation would be the child's grandmother, aunt, or other close relative. Many mothers use a day care center or shared baby-sitter. If we can afford it, an exclusive baby-sitter or nanny who comes to our home might be the best solution. We have to feel confident that the baby-sitter will provide love as well as sanitary care, but we also have to feel confident that the baby-sitter is not usurping our child's affection for mommy right there under our own roof.

Judith Klein commented that it is not unusual for the mother to be jealous of the loving relationship being developed between her baby and the sitter. If this does happen, one antidote would be to encourage the baby-sitter to attend a mother-infant playgroup, so her time together with the child is not so exclusive. The kind of personality we choose for a full-time baby-sitter is also very important. The *fit* has to be right for the mother. Some mothers prefer a grandmotherly type, who they feel will dote on the baby and yet not substitute for mommy. Others prefer a motherly woman, who in effect mothers and supports the working mother herself. Others prefer to work with a younger girl, with whom they have the sense of being in control.

Marsha H. finally opted for a younger girl as her nanny. She hired a college-trained nursery nurse, who knew that this was her *job*. "She is not a substitute for me. I told her from the beginning, 'I don't work because I don't want to be with Jason, but for other reasons. You have to fit in with my routine, and my wishes.' She talks to Jason about me a lot during the day, and they come to the window to watch me come home in the car. I feel pretty comfortable about it now."

Whether we have childcare in the home or out will depend on how much we can afford, space at home, and on our own schedule. Childcare out of the home demands a regular work routine and ease of transportation to and fro. If childcare is giving us too much stress, we will always be rushing: watching the clock, hurrying from work, worrying that the bus or subway or traffic conditions will make us late, feeling exhausted as we trek home with the baby or preschooler to face the prospect of cooking an evening meal and getting the child to bed before collapsing ourselves. We make ourselves vulnerable to PPD.

We should also watch out for demands the child may make, indicating that a change in the care situation might be necessary. By eighteen months to two years, if we are using a baby-sitter in the home, a toddler may be feeling bored and lacking company. The baby-sitter may not like to get out and about as much as we would, may not sit in the park or join playgroups with stimulating activities. If we find ourselves worrying that a toddler is bored, it will be time for a change. A sitter's hours or routine can be changed. A playgroup or, if the child is two and a half to three years old, a morning nursery school can alleviate the boredom and break up the routine, so the sitter is only picking the child up for the afternoons.

A child's crying may be more than manipulative behavior designed to induce *more* guilt in the working mother. It can also be a warning that he or she has outgrown the situation, is feeling the stress we are under. Maybe the child is being understimulated or overtired, is not getting individual attention, or is feeling lonely or rejected. We don't have to give up working but we may have to rethink and reform the schedule.

We will have guilt about leaving a child with an alternate care giver, that goes without saying, but we can check, and double-check, that everything is being done for the best. Childcare is going to cost us up to a half of our salary (if not more). Yet the answer might even be to spend a little more. If it eases our stress and makes the child more comfortable, it will be worth it in the end.

Chapter 11

PROFESSIONAL AND EXECUTIVE WOMEN

Surely successful women are not special cases for suffering PPD? You may believe, as do so many of the women in question *before* they become mothers, that these women are all set to be the new superwomen of our society. They are used to achievement, organizing, and dealing with people and situations. They have status in the working world, probably can negotiate for time off or easier working hours more successfully than a woman with a less flexible job; even better, they have money and can afford good childcare, thereby alleviating some of the guilt. What could they possibly have to complain about?

"We think we can handle anything because we're older and have advanced in our careers. Yet when we take home a tiny infant and realize the baby is totally dependent on us for everything, it's just overwhelming," marveled Suzette S., who, at thirty-six, had a fine career in banking, and was by now the mother of two small daughters. Suzette had been married for eight years before having a child and felt she was ready for anything. "But I was sure wrong!"

Some of those very qualities I have enumerated can make the

transition from professional or executive woman into working mother much harder than anyone would have imagined.

Dr. Elisabeth Herz has seen a lot of professionals in her practice. Just as Suzette disarmingly admitted, career women do not always find the path to motherhood and career as primrose-lined as they had fondly imagined. As Dr. Herz sees it, the professional or executive woman has left behind much of the conventional role of women just to get where she is. Becoming a mother pulls her back to a more traditional role: "They have learned to see themselves as different kinds of women; yet once they have been pregnant, given birth, and nursed a baby, they know they are just like other women—and yet they are *not.*" The career woman often has no role model for her type of work, the long hours, the dedication and loyalty demanded by her job or company. She has no role model for this new kind of motherhood either. The result may be a woman caught between opposing demands.

Inadequacy, often felt by new mothers, can hit the successful, organized, career woman hard. Used to being in control, meeting deadlines, working under pressure, pleasing her boss, she is not accustomed to dealing with a baby who will not sleep or will not be satisfied, or to dealing with the encroaching fears about her own identity or sanity. Isolated from other women, she seems to be neither a real professional nor a real mother.

Judith Klein commented: "Career women have long identified their work as a major source of gratification. Once they are mothers they no longer feel that same gratification toward the job itself; something else is pulling at their attention. Also, the gratification they are used to feeling at work is not so easily found in caring for an infant. There are no thank you's, no good reports, no salary increases, no boss popping his or her head around the door to say, 'Well done.' "

Laura: Career Woman, Mommy, or Neither?

By the age of thirty-three, Laura S. was so used to her career in management with an industrial firm that she approached her pregnancy and impending motherhood just as she would a management project. She handled her pregnancy well, buying the right executive pregnancy clothes, attending exercise and Lamaze classes, not putting on too much weight. She obviously had not a clue what having a baby would really be like.

"I worked to the day before delivery, everything went fine. I thought I'd covered my tracks well as a corporate woman. I even scheduled to go in for a couple of meetings a week after the birth, imagining I'd be able to leave the baby with my mother—after all, what's a kid? I had no idea. Nobody anywhere, in Lamaze classes or any of the books, told me, 'Hey, wait a minute. I don't mean to be scary but there's no way you'll be able to go in to the office the first week after giving birth.' It was a nightmare for me.

"I'm a career woman. Yet I started thinking of myself as a mommy. I'm with a very male-oriented company and no one expected me to come back. Those middle-management guys have wives back home in the suburbs and feel a woman's place is at home with the kids. It's even been depressing for me at work, because I find I'm more 'female' now. I get upset and confused, want to cry. I think about Bobby when I should be thinking about work. Being at home and depressed would be helplessness, but this is hopelessness, because I can't do anything right. Bobby is up at nights, and I have a business meeting in the morning. I've never been this emotional before."

One of Laura's problems had been the lack of support she found from other women. Having moved to the suburbs before they started their family, Laura discovered herself isolated in that community, surrounded by stay-at-home mothers. She hunted for a support group either in the suburban area or in the city where she worked, anything that would bring together a group of women *after office hours.* When we met, Laura had been unable to find any such group.

The books on childcare, she pointed out, aim at stay-at-home mothers. "They tell you what to expect each month of your child's development. 'This is the month the child finally falls in love with you, you're the number-one person,' they read. I have a live-in baby-sitter, and I read this section and thought, 'Great, now Bobby is going to fall in love with Lynn. He spends most of his time with her.' " Laura's identity problem was acute.

Perhaps this was the real clue to her mental distress. The mere fact that she went back to the office for some meetings the week after childbirth would not in itself create a problem. (Laura returned to full-time work after six weeks.) Many women have found getting straight back into office life, if only for one or two days a week, of great help in adjusting to motherhood, and to working motherhood—it has meant not losing touch with their work and their colleagues, thus avoiding being cast in the role of outsider, which women necessarily worry about in today's competitive world.

As we learned in the section on breast-feeding, Laura had first had a problem with the image of herself as a mother. She had quickly lost excess weight after childbirth but had been unable to breast-feed. She had serious doubts about her femininity, which emerged in the acute sense of isolation she felt living in the suburbs, surrounded by stay-at-home mothers, commuting to the city for work, where she was surrounded by male colleagues at her level.

Laura's PPD was evident to herself and to her husband, Nick. But, at the time we met, she had found no help from doctors or books and continued to feel mild despair. She could get by, she said. Her work was not suffering, but her marriage was showing the strains, and her relationship with five-month-old Bobby was still tense. Physically, Laura's PPD could have been evident to doctors too, from the first few days after birth when the milk did not come into her breasts. The hormone prolactin was not being released in sufficient quantities. Her endocrinological system was not flourishing or functioning as it should. One other physical symptom was that even at five months after childbirth, and without breast-feeding, Laura's hair was falling out. If only more were generally understood about PPD, this rather sad young woman would not have had to undergo such a long, lonely time of distress.

THE DRIVE FOR PERFECTION

Executive women put heavy demands on themselves to be perfect. But if they expect to be perfect as professionals and as mothers, they will not succeed at either. Worse, the dissatisfaction with themselves if they fail the "perfect" test can lead to breakdown. Dr. Herz emphasized three main realities executive women should bear in mind to ease this destructive drive:

1. They may fall behind in their careers in the early years of their children's lives. They may not be as good at work nor be able to earn promotions or raises, because drive and ambition will likely decline due to simple exhaustion, primary satisfaction in mothering, or other factors.
2. They will have to hire help, probably full time, unless they happen to have a husband whose hours are flexible enough to take a major role in childcare.
3. They will not be available to their children as and when they might wish they could be.

These realities, if ignored, may result in an unwarranted sense of guilt when a woman faces her lack of energy for coping with husband, child, and career.

TOO SELF-CRITICAL

The more high-powered, the more successful a woman is in her career, the harder she may find adjustment to mothering. Dr. Herz pinpointed another cause of distress that may lead to serious PPD, which any professional mother should consider.

Professional women tend to be compulsive and overly conscientious. They need this personality trait to have achieved their position. Used to striving for perfection and generally quite self-critical, they are—Dr. Herz perceives—too negative and unrealistic in their self-evaluations.

"The gap between a woman's unrealistically idealized image of mother and career woman and her overcritical assessment of what she is may be very great. The wider the gap the worse she feels. What may follow is a total loss of self-confidence with a quick slide into depression. It's one of the dynamics we see over and over again."

Sara G., a thirty-six-year-old lawyer had been delighted to have her first baby, although in retrospect she suffered a slight depression that had been camouflaged by returning immediately to work, with full-time help, continuing to lead a very active life, and becoming pregnant again shortly after. The second baby was born eighteen months later.

After this second birth, Sara's depression was overwhelming. It was not picked up by her doctor or obstetrician. It was quite a while before she was referred to one of the small band of psychosomatic ob/gyns available. By this time, although still at work, Sara was almost nonfunctional, with a severe sleep disorder, and her work had reached a nonproductive end. Her sense of self-worth was practically nonexistent. She had begun to overeat, and the weight problem was only worsening her low self-esteem.

Sara was started on a course of antidepressants while working closely with a psychiatrist for three months to deal with the lowered self-esteem and confused identity. Discussing a case like this, Dr. Herz explained, "Sadly, some psychiatrists are not really tuned into PPD. They delve too far into the past. I believe we need to know something about a woman's background and her responses and defenses to previous crises, but not necessarily to explore childhood conflicts and relationships.

"The mixture of antidepressants and short-term therapy can be very successful. I will talk to a woman, and when she begins to berate herself, I say, 'Well, tell me what you did yesterday.' When she lists all the things she has accomplished, I point out that she has been doing a lot, and an awful lot very well. But she cannot see it. We discuss in detail what sort of compromises she might be able to make in her own life, either with work or mothering, that would ease the burden."

The professional or executive woman is especially vulnerable to PPD. Because she is used to success and keeping her life in control, a sense of failure or of emotional extremes can be too hard to deal with. In the past, she might have sought a solution in handing the child over to a full-time nanny, returning to the safe security of her own work, and escaping the problems. But today, with more enlightened and concerned care available to her, she can resolve her problems with greater insight.

BUSINESS TRIPS OR TIME AWAY ON YOUR OWN

Can the professional woman safely, or justifiably, take time away from her child—anything from three days to two weeks—to go on a business trip, attend a sales conference, go on a brief vacation, or simply have some time to think and be alone? Women's views on this question will vary, depending on the amount of guilt already felt about leaving the child during the work day, the amount of support received from the husband or other close family, and the mother's own feelings of separation from her child. Another variable will be the level of her ambition or concern about competition within her company.

In my own life, if possible, I travel without my children for a four- to ten-day period each year to give myself some free time in which to pursue business, meet with friends, make necessary contacts, and let that old childless identity breathe again. I doubt I would go for any longer than that brief interlude, during which, I hope, the children have scarcely had time to accept that I am gone before I am back again. Sometimes I find myself imagining, however, that the high-powered career woman who dashes off to three-day conferences or takes important sales trips finds it easier to leave her child with her full-time housekeeper, easier to justify that she must go for her work; easier at least than being forced to admit, *"I am doing this for myself. Time away from motherhood is good for me; helps me put my new life in perspective."*

The question begs other ones: how do we blend ambition and career with the pressures and concerns of motherhood? Or, *Who is going to sacrifice whose life to whom?* Does motherhood have to equal self-sacrifice?

I have in mind a young actress, married to another actor. While their baby, Ben, was an infant, Carrie D. tended to stay home, but she never forgot her desire to succeed in the theater, which had been as strong as her husband's. They lived in a major city near potential work. But, as luck would have it, her husband, Don, landed a great part in a repertory company five hundred miles away. He took the job, and Carrie was left on her own bringing up Ben for stretches as long as three months at a time.

There was not enough money to pay airfares back and forth any more often than perhaps once during the three-month separations.

Ben went to nursery school, and I used to see Carrie looking not exactly depressed but not elated, either. She was hunting for work but finding it hard going. Then I didn't see her for a while. Ben was being picked up from school by a baby-sitter. Eventually I heard that Carrie had landed work—as luck would have it, just like her husband—outside of the city. It was not as far away as Don's company, but in a small town an hour's ride away. Carrie had to stay out of town three nights a week, rushing home the other four. "Who looks after Ben?" was my first thought. They had a baby-sitter sleep over those three nights. "Does he mind?" I asked my source. She laughed. "Ben's an independent, feisty little boy. I have him over to play sometimes after school. It strikes me now that all this stuff about staying home with your kids is nonsense. Carrie brought Ben up to be independent. He's used to dealing with both his parents' absences. He knows she'll be back. Acting is important to Carrie and I think she was right not to turn that work down, even though her husband is out of town too. It's not easy getting acting jobs!"

We make our own decisions based on our blend of ambition, guilt, fear of harming the child, desire to raise an independent child who respects his or her mother's work, and availability of the father or perhaps a grandmother to help out in our absence. We no doubt take the advice of pediatricians and child psychologists and digest the material we wish or are prepared to hear on whether they feel it is safe to leave an infant, a toddler, a two-year-old, three-year-old, etc.

The infant is the easiest to leave for short periods, as long as you are not breast-feeding. Good loving alternative care can be given without the child even knowing mother is not there. Toddlers from a year to two years can be very difficult to leave behind: their emotions are so outward and so passionate that it may be heart-wrenching to witness the pain of their separation. Even three-year-olds who speak well may be quick to pierce the heart with pleas not to be abandoned. But the decision, ultimately, must lie with the individual rather than with what society feels is best. Her work, her need to make that particular trip, her personal development and need for space and time are all as important considerations as is the welfare of the child. Mother counts too.

If you have a grandparent or another close relative nearby, the best solution to your absence would probably be to pay for outside help in the home (so you are not expecting granny to do all the work) and then invite the relative to your house as a *treat* for the child and as a buffer zone of stability and security in your place.

WEEKEND MOTHERING

One of our much-loved images of working mothers is that they miss their children so badly all day and all week, they long for weekends so they can spend precious time with them. That notion may be the stuff of fairy tales and tends to negate the very real personal needs of mothers and fathers. If we have worked five days, if we have lived by the clock and schedule, come the weekend we crave some time to ourselves. Time to catch up on laundry and household work, buy clothes or birthday presents or groceries; do some cooking for the week ahead, take exercise classes or play tennis, or simply get together with friends or relatives. How do we find that time?

Weekends are also for marriages, for spending time together as husband and wife, for love and socializing, and even for sex! As parents we yearn for those lazy weekends devoted to self-indulgent pursuits. So why not admit it? Now that we are parents thoughts about weekends tend to be, "How can we best entertain the child, get some time to ourselves together, and allow time off individually?"

Even Jeanne N., with her live-in help on alternate weekends, furrowed her brow at the question of weekends. I imagined her life must be a dream compared to most. "Oh, no, they're really hard on us as a couple," she said. "There is no rest or peace. I see my husband very little during the week, with our busy schedules, and although the housekeeper might take the children out to the park for an hour or so, basically we're there with the kids.

"I usually have a lot of reading to catch up on, maybe manuscripts to be worked on, authors to talk to. My husband wants to relax, play tennis. I plead with him that I have work to do. I see that look of frustration in his eyes."

We can all think of one or two women who seem to combine successfully a position as corporate vice president with a happy marriage, one or two children, and the roles of stunning cook, hostess, and interior decorator as well. But a normal human being does not have the energy, emotional strength, or intellectual tenacity to cope perfectly with career, deal lovingly with her husband, give to her children the amount of love and time they, or she, would like, and spend time on domestic duties that suit her self-image as a woman.

We have to accept our own limitations, and some unwelcome compromises. If we don't, we will be leaving ourselves vulnerable to PPD brought on by exhaustion and an overcritical judgment of ourselves that everything we do is a failure. The psychological and the physiological march in tandem for the professional and executive woman as they do for any other mother. Believing she can do everything, refusing to see the need for compromise, and denying the real psychological impact of the lack of role models for her type of mothering can all too quickly lead a driven woman to total collapse and severe PPD.

Chapter 12

WORKING AT HOME

COMPROMISE OR CHOSEN PATH?

A woman's self-image helps program her for this kind of compromise. In my own life, fantasies had never included myself as a housewife and mother or as a high-powered executive mother. The road to my compromise was plotted long before I had a baby, following some preconceived blueprint of acceptable female behavior that was less consciously worked out than achieved by instinct. I gave up a well-paid, interesting newspaper job in my late twenties to become a freelance home-based writer. Maintaining to the outside world that I had made the bold move because I needed to force myself into insecurity to become a real writer, I also had secret reasons I did not brag about to colleagues or friends.

In the not-so-distant future, though I was not yet married and showed little sign of ever being so, I wanted to be a mother. When I had a child, I would want to be at home, as my mother had always been, to greet my young family coming in from school. Unlike my mother, I knew I would want to keep up my work and felt I should get started now, to be ready when the day came. I was, in effect, feathering the nest.

In my fantasies, you notice, I had conveniently omitted the first five or six years before a child even goes to school to be so warmly greeted home again by the smell of freshly baked cookies. So much for fantasies. Nor had I sat down with a calculator and forecast the cost of childcare and the possibility of my work as a writer being able to fund such a luxurious way of life. Ultimately, however, it has been a good compromise for me.

I can feel like a real mother, yet I am not totally stuck at home. I know that I would hate spending all day, every day, with my children. I am not God's gift to motherhood, have little patience, get easily bored, and do not want to spend my days helping my daughters cut and paste. On the good days, I work contentedly at home, and when the baby-sitter brings my youngest one home from nursery school, we stop to chat before going on with our separate functions.

When the children were younger I had no formal baby-sitting routine, as I was not earning enough to justify the cost. Determinedly I enforced a nap routine and *stole* two or more hours a day in which to work. I craved that time, needed to impose the regimen. My mind needed the freedom and liberty of concentration and focused thought. Any work acts as a tremendous release from the strains of motherhood. Just two hours of concentrated thought on some project of my own, on adult concepts, seemed to be enough to repair the ravages left by dealing with young children.

There is more to it than that. My freelance work gets me out of the house. I meet other adults (not necessarily mothers) and get to talk about things dear to my heart (other than toilet training). Some days are great fun, racing around researching a topic and coming home to my children. Other days are a plain hard grind, working all day at the typewriter, not daring to take time to read the newspaper, or talk to a friend, or indulge myself at all, then having to make dinner and deal with the children. At the end of my working day, the farthest I have to walk is from study to kitchen, there to meet two cranky children, who have to be fed, bathed, listened to, loved, played with, and argued with, and finally put to bed. And then, oh joy, I get to baby-sit for them and maybe snatch a few hours' more work in the evening. Those are the bad days.

Is working at home really a compromise between the working world and the mothering world? Those women who have taken the option feel they are getting some of the best of both worlds. They are perhaps instinctively, as I can see in myself, avoiding various levels of potential threats of PPD: avoiding the role and identity confusion of the full-time or executive working mother, her exhaustion and inability to find time for all the priorities in her life; and avoiding the traps of loss of identity, loss of financial independence, and the gradual mental vegetation of many stay-at-home mothers who have little outlet for release or escape.

I am not implying that all working mothers should make such a compromise. As the New York *Times Magazine* article "The Working Mother as Role Model," referred to earlier, has shown, babies and young children of full-time working mothers seem to be more than usually alert and contented, either in day care or with an alternative care giver, and they are socially active and perform well on adaptive-skills tests. Perhaps this is so because they have *two* stimulating parents. (Though I beg to differ with the implication that stay-at-home mothers, by definition, are nurturing, warm, and *non*stimulating!) In my daughter's nursery school, this conversation between two four-year-old girls was reported: discussing what they wanted to be as grown-ups, one replied, "Oh, I don't want to be a lawyer. All mommies do that. It's boring."

WHY THE COMPROMISE SOMETIMES FAILS

Working at home notoriously does not pay well; there are no benefits, no sick pay, no holiday pay, and precious little in the way of status or prestige (unless you get lucky). For the ambitious or career-minded it is therefore often very much a compromise, taken in an effort to fit more mothering and less daily work into their lives. Unfortunately, the situation many women find themselves in, once they become mothers, is not really being sure what they want out of the working world and what they feel they should put in. Then the compromise seems to fail, for these women will not feel adequately rewarded either financially or in terms of status. I doubt their choice of work by itself leads to PPD; their confusion was already strong enough to set off depression.

Ellen C. is such a woman. A former lawyer, now turned forty, with two nearly school-age children, she told me she only gave up work because she could not make up her mind whether she really wanted to continue in a full-time lawyer's position or whether she wanted to be home with her new baby. When her first child was six months old, she did quit her job, anxious and paranoid that the sitter she had hired was mistreating her baby. The second baby came within the next year, and suddenly Ellen found that a free decision had become cemented as a way of life. "But I certainly was not made to be a housewife. So I drifted into part-time legal work that I could do from home. I cannot say I am happy, no. I don't any longer know what would make me happy. Going back full-time into a prosecutor's office would not be the answer. But then neither is this stateless, nameless sort of position I hold right now."

Ellen admits that her depression is a chronic but mild one that has become the predominant feature of her life. Whatever germ of PPD set in, in those first few weeks after the baby's birth, has never lifted. Ellen feels out of control of her life. She resents her husband's earning power. Even the fact that they can afford to pay for private schools and Ellen contributes nothing toward that expense makes her feel she accomplishes nothing. "My husband is as good at dealing with the children as I am. He doesn't do more because he has to be out of the house. So where does that leave me? I'm pretty much a nobody these days."

As for Ellen's freelance legal work, for which she has been able to convert a basement into an office, she finds it unsatisfactory because of the long hours spent for little compensation, when she is fully aware how much lawyers can demand in the outside world.

"Also, I don't have a decompression chamber like my husband does. I may cut myself off from the children, who are brought home by the sitter, to be entertained by her until I'm finished for the day. But it means I walk straight from the office, up the stairs, to deal with arguing, crying, hungry kids. I get angry at my husband again at those times, wondering why he never gets home early enough to take over those duties. But then how many husbands do?"

Chapter 13

STAY-AT-HOME MOTHERS

Why do some mothers choose to stay home with their children? That may be a strange question in a world where society is still pushing the importance of that very option, still critical of women who do work once they are mothers. For many women that is the only choice. Maybe as little girls, teenagers, young adult women seeking love and partnership, they saw themselves in the image of full-time nurturing mother. They promised themselves that when they had a baby they would give up working, if only for five years or so.

Once they are mothers, they know a child needs them around, just as their mothers were around for them (or, if not, as they dreamed their mothers would be). They intend to give their child the best possible start in life. They do not trust leaving their baby with a stranger. They would never use day care centers because they believe it is the parents' duty to raise their own children. Who else could possibly give the love needed to their child? Husband, mother, close friends, all expected them to give up working and to do the right thing by the child.

There may be financial reasons for this choice as well. The sort of work many women are involved in does not cover the cost of baby-sitting or alternative care, or does not interest them sufficiently to offer an alternative to mothering as a way of life.

Thankfully, fewer and fewer women are feeling out of control over the decision. Somehow they blend the various forces at work into a valid credo for living. In my own urban neighborhood, the majority of women seem to have opted for full-time motherhood. These are not young girls in their early twenties, with not a clue as to what they are doing or why. For the most part they are women in their late twenties and early to late thirties.

I see them as the "class of '68." There they are, chatting with one another in the playground, content to pass their days entertaining one or two muddied preschool children. Their days are domestically oriented, organized around the child's program rather than theirs. Yet they are not complaining; they are not characters from Marilyn French's *The Women's Room;* they don't feel they are suffering from insensitive husbands who have no idea what their day or routine is like. They don't feel they have sacrificed their career for their husband's, nor do they feel unduly exploited. Content and at ease with the decision to drop the joys of working for the joys of motherhood, they feel perhaps an extra layer of contentment in a deeply rooted aura of self-righteousness.

Stay-at-home mothers as a cultural group tend to be on the defensive about their image and lifestyle choice. One of the saddest outcomes of this flight behind the barriers of self-defense is that full-time mothers have little understanding of or sympathy for working mothers, and vice versa. The two sides appear to be so firmly entrenched in their own dogma that they might be at war. "If you go to work, why have a child in the first place? You never get to see your child during the day, so why become a mother?" argue the stay-at-homes. "They have no identity, they'll be stuck in a few years' time with no work, no money, and their husbands will leave them. What's so great about staying home, when all I see in the supermarkets is these women yelling at their kids or hitting them?" argue the working mothers.

SOME JUST AREN'T SUITED TO STAYING HOME

Stay-at-home mothers have a lot of emotional investment in their mothering, and denial that anything might be wrong is strong in their psyches. PPD can strike stay-at-home mothers as fiercely, if not more so, than any other woman. Worse, their symptoms are more likely to go unchecked as, culturally, they are expected to suffer or react this way and, financially, have not the wherewithal to seek professional help.

Many women who make the choice to be full-time mothers may, along the way, realize it was not the right decision for them. This change of self-image can be hard to reconcile with that self-righteousness. Such mothers may find themselves locked in a resentful, hostile battle with their husbands, expressed either in sexual jealousy or envy of his advancement at work and his comparatively glamorous life. Others may sink into swift decline, finding the cabbage-patch mentality taking them over like an invader from outer space.

When Nancy E., for example, was twenty-five years old and had her first daughter, she had been ecstatic at being a full-time mother. "I just wasn't cut out to be a working mother. At first I had to go back to teaching, for the money, but every moment of my baby's development was too precious to share with someone else. So I gave up teaching and, to take in extra money, I started baby-sitting for friends. I loved taking care of infants, and never had any problems."

When Nancy had the second baby, at age thirty-one, she discovered she had changed in the intervening years in ways she did not recognize. She no longer wanted to be a full-time mother and housewife. This reversal contradicted everything she had ever believed about herself, from the days of playing with dolls and waiting to grow up to be a mommy.

"I had always seen myself as a typical housewife, baking bread, cleaning the house, making cookies. But then it dawned on me, after the second child, that I *hate* housework. I just didn't want to go back to all that."

Immediately after the baby, she felt confined to the house

again, after years of working with her husband in their own business, Nancy said, "I still believed women were supposed to be home with their children, so my picture of myself just didn't fit any more. Yet I also knew I needed something more. I needed my work." Nancy, as we saw earlier, suffered a severe PPD. Her road out of that crisis was partly smoothed by a shared decision with her husband that she would go back into the business two days a week. The treatment she received from the psychiatrist, antidepressant medication, alone would not have shifted the PPD. It took time and honest talking with her husband before she began to fit the pieces together and learn that some of the strain on her psyche had been imposed by her own idealized fantasy of herself as a full-time mother, which just did not fit the reality of her life nearly a decade later.

A MOVE BEYOND TOTAL MOTHERHOOD

PPD may be a sign for some women that they need to branch out in a wider direction, away from total motherhood. Lucy C. was another example of just those forces of change. At twenty-six, after the birth of her second child, following just fifteen months after the first, Lucy expected some weepiness and was prepared for it. She was content with her decision to be home with the children, yet she fell into a severe depression. She was unable to get out of bed in the morning: just getting through the day was hard. Fortunately for her, an eighty-year-old aunt came to stay, and it was the aunt who suggested that, first, Lucy should see a doctor about her depression, and second, maybe she should consider doing something more with her life.

Lucy felt foolish and weak after seeing the doctor, because he implied that her depression was symptomatic of a more severe psychiatric disorder. Lucy dismissed out of hand the idea of seeing a psychotherapist. Finally, however, at her aunt's insistence, she did begin seeing a therapist *and* she went back to school to get her master's degree. The aunt offered to stay for a few weeks, to baby-sit, until Lucy got herself sorted out. Oh, that we could all have such wise and supportive relatives!

"If anyone had told me it would take ten months to shift the

PPD after the birth of my son, I would have laughed in their face," Lucy later commented. She had imagined motherhood would be easy. But the full-time commitment had dragged her down, to a status she hardly recognized in herself.

SICKNESS AND SNOWY DAYS: PRISONER TO THE HOME

Whether we are stay-at-home or working mothers, the advent of a heavy snow or a child's sickness, meaning we have to stay home for a day or more, may renew in any of us the entrapment feeling of early PPD. No amount of logic ("It's only a day or so out of a lifetime") seems to banish that fear of being a prisoner in our own homes. The sheer pressure of the huge responsibility can suffocate us, and any notion of freedom or "I've got it all sorted out now" may vanish once the snow or sickness sets in.

Often sick as a child, I hated to discover in myself as a mother a total intolerance and impatience with my elder daughter, who seemed to have inherited my feeble genes almost deliberately to punish me.

Yet my own memories of childhood illnesses are pleasant. I would lie in bed surrounded by toys and coloring books my father would bring home as a special treat in the evenings; my mother would carry carefully thought-out meals to my sickbed and sit with me through the afternoons, reading stories.

Why couldn't I be like that? What had happened to that image of myself as the nuturing-caring-giving mother? There I was again, sliding away from my image of perfect mother.

I am thirty-eight years old and, until recently, it had never occurred to me that my mother might also have resented my sick days. How did she manage something as simple as getting out to buy food? How did her identity hold up under house arrest? I finally asked her and, yes, she hated it, too. She had longed for weekends, when my father would be home and she could leave me, if only to go shopping, anything to get out of the house.

Nancy E. also described complete mood reversals once she was snowed in.

"When I was a child, there were three of us, and my mother

often had us all sick at home. My father did nothing to help her. I remember my mother looking like she would drop. On those days she never went out of the house, she dedicated everything to us. I'm not sure if our mothers didn't do us an injustice. I don't think it was good for us to see such self-sacrifice to children, being so totally selfless. When we try and become a mother in that image, that's when we come unstuck," she explained.

We do feel resentment when our sick child needs us most, and we can't help but feel guilty about that. As a self-employed worker, I fear the encroachment of my work time. Will I ever get the project finished? Will my career ever get anywhere? Will I justify the cost of childcare by making enough money?

Part-time working mothers are vulnerable to instant firing if they take too many days off because a child is sick. Full-time working mothers have enormous problems if they rely on a day care center and their child is often out sick or if they rely on a baby-sitter who is herself off sick too many times. Huge rows flare up between husbands and wives; moral debates over who is going to take the day off; who is going to incur the wrath of the boss, risk losing a promotion, risk loss of pay, make the sacrifice.

There is no way around it. Sick days and snow days reemphasize some of the negative aspects of mothering, or the negative aspects of ourselves as mothers. Where is the saint we imagined we would be? And hello again guilt and recrimination, which might set off another bout of PPD, once we felt clear of the despondency.

THERE IS NO SUCH THING AS A FREE LUNCH

For me the involvement of motherhood can best be summed up in that phrase.

It came from a lunch date I had organized with a fellow (childless) writer. Both self-employed and working in our separate homes, we used to meet once a month to gossip, trade notes, and bitch about late payments and rejected manuscripts. But now I had two small children, and to get out for lunch meant arranging a baby-sitter.

Hold on, I said to myself, it is going to cost as much for the sitter as for the lunch, and add to that the transport, plus the fact that it will eat up three hours of my day, and they would be the only "free" hours (paid for and free of children), which would be better served by my working, not lunching.

Now was the time to schedule my available money, who my friends would be, and how I would make ultimate use of the energy levels—and material resources—that realistically I knew existed, not the ones I dreamed of having.

When a woman has a child, unless she has a very helpful husband, mother, or neighbor, any free time will be paid, negotiated for, or traded off against. To go to the hairdresser, dentist, doctor, health club, swimming pool, department store, church, or to do some work—even if the time is just to be alone and think—she will have to pay for it in some fashion.

PART FOUR

Helping Ourselves, Helping Each Other

Chapter 14

A GAME PLAN FOR SURVIVAL

Most new mothers would prefer to think they could avoid PPD altogether, with some carefully prepared plan of survival; or that if signs of depression begin to set in that they would know what steps are best taken to prevent it worsening. We have to go right back to basics for any such plan and really think out how we are going to prevent biochemical upheaval from taking over our lives. If the body's and the brain's hormones find the way of life just too overwhelming, they will tell us—in no uncertain manner (even if we had not already got the intensity of the message ourselves)—that it is time for a change.

The self-help techniques I am going to discuss can, advisably, help only those women whose symptoms of PPD are mild or moderate and that come on slowly, with no exaggerated danger signals involved. Any woman who is undergoing suicidal fantasies or fears she might harm her baby should not waste her time trying to pull herself together but must seek good professional help immediately. Unfortunately, the extreme variety of PPD, which usually comes on within the first two weeks after childbirth, symptoms of which are intense and frightening, tends to be completely out of our control and should not be dealt with lightly.

MILD TO MODERATE PPD

Let us look first at the best approach to PPD for the 10 percent of new mothers statistically reported to suffer what we would ourselves describe as mild to moderate symptoms. (In my view the figure is much higher, as very few in this group actually seek professional help).

The best and most immediate help might come in the form of someone genuinely sympathetic to talk to. That listener may be our husband, a friend who has been there and will admit it, or a counselor or psychotherapist whom we seek out or to whom we have been referred by a concerned obstetrician or family doctor. Parents' or mothers' support groups are of great help for those with mild to moderate PPD, offering us a chance to compare notes, put all the new stresses and burdens in perspective, and share a few laughs.

WHERE ARE YOU FINDING YOUR BASIC RESOURCES?

Any new mother should sit down, preferably with her husband, and begin to discuss where she (or he) is finding her resources and energy levels now that they have a baby. You need to be aware of (a) sleep and adequate rest; (b) time for yourself (and himself) and for yourselves as a couple; (c) money; and (d) stimulating interests outside your new life as parents.

Ideally, a lot of this work would have been done before the baby was born. But it is still a fantasy to imagine couples really facing seriously the problems they might have to overcome once they are parents. However, a prenatal plan can be followed if you have previously suffered PPD and are determined to avoid it this time. For those couples, I would say, forget the buying of crib and diapers, forget the lessons on breathing and relaxation for labor and delivery, and concern yourselves right now with the fundamental life changes and the effects they might have on both of you.

THE PRENATAL PLAN

1. Accept that PPD can easily follow the birth of any child and adopt a nonjudgmental attitude toward yourself. The basis of PPD is hormonal and neurohormonal; it is not an indication of your failure. You should not feel guilt, shame, or fear at unexpected emotional reactions to yourself as a mother or to your baby. You should expect to go through some ambivalence about becoming a mother and toward your baby.
2. Talk to your husband about the possibility of PPD and what you will do in the event; i.e., think of alternate sources of help, face the question of who will look after the baby if you have to get twenty-four hours of sleep or enter a hospital for care. Encourage your husband to appreciate his role as a partner and make sure he understands that you cannot be *expected* to cope with everything.
3. Discuss your attitude to breast-feeding and whether you feel capable of the very real emotional, psychological, and physical drain of full-time nursing. Discuss the idea with your husband of giving your baby one bottle a day so he can share in some of the duties and give you a chance to catch up on sleep, or take time out alone from the baby.
4. Discuss how you are both going to get time to yourselves. Check out baby-sitting arrangements in your area. Would your husband give up one evening a week regularly so you could go out? Would your mother or mother-in-law help? If not, how will you pay for the time? Discuss the costs of childcare and baby-sitting now, and *save*.
5. Try and summarize your lifestyle by writing a list of what you would really miss if it were to be changed. Run through your own index of independence, desire for freedom, sociability, the significance of hobbies or exercise to you, the need for privacy, and the amount of time you are used to spending alone, with friends, and with other adults.

   Imagine yourself under house arrest and underline what you would miss most. Get your husband to do the same. Work together on how you would fit those needs into a new life. If you were used to working all day, exercising after work, meeting friends one evening a week, and your husband was used to going out one evening and sports on a weekend day, what can you *both* give up? Could you trade off two evenings for you against a weekend day for him?

6. If you plan to return to full-time work, don't think only about childcare arrangements, think about *you.* Try to listen very carefully to your heart and head, to your personal contentment level, right now, not only in the job itself but in being out and about in the day, in deriving pleasure from colleagues and in earning your own salary. It is difficult to know whether you should plan to return to work immediately, perhaps for one or two days a week, plan for a minimum of three months' leave, or six months' (taking leave without pay to spend more time with your newborn). But it is a vital decision to your ultimate ease in adjusting to working motherhood.

   Keep your options open if you are unsure (and even if you aren't). Don't brag too much about how you are going to hate going back to work, knowing you'll be so happy at home with the baby. Many women have found they returned to work earlier than they had planned because they could not deal with encroaching PPD symptoms and feeling tied down in the house.

   Try and talk to some other women at work who have recently had babies, and see if they would be interested in setting up a working mothers' group. Suggest you could meet once every three to four weeks for lunch and to compare complaints, tips, or problems with childcare.

7. Talk to your husband about the change in salary if you are taking a leave of absence. What will one salary mean to both of you? What about the cost of childcare? Could you manage domestic help when you return to work, someone to help out with shopping, laundry, cleaning? Would a baby-sitter who would come to the house and do light chores be easier than day care for you?

8. *Keep your options open* if you are planning not to return to work. You'll never know what you will feel about full-time

motherhood until you try it first-hand. Keep some contact with the workplace because you may feel like going back, even half a day a week, or mornings only; or you might change your mind altogether and want to return full time. If you are going to work at home, check out childcare arrangements now and talk to your husband about the need to have some alternate care system worked out, even if you are not fully earning to cover those costs. Accept that you will not be as productive nor able to keep your income at the same level with a child as you were alone, however much you fantasize being skillful at both.

9. Don't get too carried away on the romance and joy of motherhood. Maybe it will come, maybe it won't.
10. What sort of support system will you have? Be honest about this. If your husband is a traditionalist and your family lives miles away, your friends are all single and devoted to wild late-night parties, is there anyone around who might feel sympathetic? Do you have anyone—close friend, husband, doctor—who is a real confidante? Someone who is not shocked by any disclosure? Has any friend with a baby ever hinted to you that everything is not all roses? She is the one to call after the birth.

    One way of trying to ensure you have support resources in the bank would be to baby-sit for a friend's new baby or young children while you are still childfree. You will accustom yourself to some of the inequities of childcare that way, and will then feel less as though you are imposing when you turn to that same friend for help, advice, reassurance—and baby-sitting—once you have your own baby.
11. Do you have overloading factors before giving birth? Spend some time thinking about your life—your desires, personal goals, and attitudes to mothering *now*. You might be able to work out some strategies that would help you achieve all your goals beforehand. Areas you should give thought to: did you delay childbirth because of ambivalence; did you have more than one therapeutic abortion; have you had several miscarriages; are there stepchildren in the household; did you have an infertility problem before this pregnancy; have

you recently moved; how well is your work going; do you have a career that you consider important; how do your self-image and confidence survive under stress or attack; have you recently lost someone you loved dearly; did your mother die when you were a child; are you used to spending a lot of time out of the house, either alone or with your husband; is your marriage new and in what experts call the erotic stage.

If you feel that any of these overloading factors might bother you later, get in touch with a counselor or therapist now and talk over some of the difficulties you might have in adjusting to motherhood.

POSTPARTUM PLAN

To avoid biochemical upheaval or psychological distress after childbirth, you will need to give time and thought to the following factors.

STRESS AND TENSION

It is too easy to be flip or patronizing with advice on avoiding stress and tension for new mothers, when the very fact of becoming a new mother provides stress and tension. You may feel zombielike most of the time, so overwhelming will be the changes to your life and life patterns, the intense emotional involvement, and the fatigue of caring for a newborn.

The worst provocation of stress, however, will not be found in the obvious strain and tiredness of infant care. Rather it will be found in the previous section, in the list of overloading factors. Any or all of these factors could be placing an undue burden on your psyche and emotional well-being, and should not be overlooked. During this period, it is advisable to talk over with your husband, or with a very close friend, any of these secret anxieties. Try not to keep up a stoic facade of "I'm coping" because you imagine that's what good mothers do. Try to rid your mind of those preconceived fantasies about what you will be like as a mother. If you don't feel warm and nurturing, but instead tense, aggravated, and resentful, confront those feelings with *someone.*

That will help release stress or tension. Accepting that you are not perfect may help you relax more into your new role.

Try to focus on what the stress is doing to *you*, rather than always worrying about its effect on the baby. The likelihood is the baby will breeze through its early months not noticing whether you are the earth-mother type or a neurotic nut-case! The baby only wants to feed and sleep and feel secure—it really does not care about your particular personality makeup at this time. As was discussed in the section on colic, your tension will not be the cause of crying in the newborn. Your inadequacy as a mother will not be the reason your baby fails to sleep through the night or seems to be fussy or cranky.

We have to learn to off-load much of the guilt we have accepted as our own in this motherhood business.

Practically, there are several ways of avoiding stress buildup, or depleting its stock once it has risen to dangerous levels. They are obvious, but often need spelling out to anxious new mothers.

SLEEP

You need sleep just as your baby needs it. Adequate sleep and rest will help prevent mental or physical exhaustion. Broken sleep cycles make the most saintly of us cranky, irritable, nervous, and unable to concentrate and can lead to depression. Broken sleep cycles have been used as an effective form of torture. An accumulation of consecutive nights without sleep may lead you to a total collapse.

Some women have found that after seven or more nights without proper sleep, they drop off on the sofa and, forgetting about the baby, sleep for eight to ten hours. The husband, mother, or friend who is in the home is then forced to take over, usually with a bottle of formula. Babies survive the emergency action, even if they are used to total breast-feeding. Mothers who can give in to their physical needs that way usually survive better, too. Women have described to me the point when they knew they could not take the sleeplessness any more. One woman told her husband he had to take over, and she checked into a local motel for the night. If such actions seem selfish to you, I suggest the opposite. It is too much self-sacrifice that leads to much distress these days. The push for total breast-feeding, on-demand schedules, has forced women to see themselves as the unimportant person in the picture. Their needs have to be denied for the baby's superior needs. That kind of attitude can lead to PPD, since we deny ourselves and in so doing obviously lose touch with our own identity and self-esteem. A little bit of selfishness is very important.

The stress and tension of a second baby, or third, when your children are close-spaced, are obviously much worse. You must pay attention to your own energy reserves—the supply is not inexhaustible. You *will* need help, to give you time to be with the infant and time to spend with the siblings, about whom you will be suffering acute guilt and anxiety at your betrayal of their needs. Accept your need for help. Make plans for friends, neighbors, family, or, failing any of those resources, talk to your husband about paying for a sitter or some form of household help. Just because women in the past always seemed able to cope does not mean you will be able to. Point out that women in the past usually lived in an extended family and therefore did have help.

If you find yourself cracking under the pressure, and your husband feels you cannot afford to pay for help, maybe you should call on your mother or mother-in-law to come and stay for a while, even if you preferred to go it alone. A few family squabbles might be worth it, if in return you were allowed a little more time to rest, and to yourself. Failing all such measures, I strongly advise that you emulate the woman mentioned in the previous paragraph. Walk out of the house and check into a motel for twenty-four hours, leaving your husband to cope. That way he might see what you mean.

BREAST-FEEDING

Try and evolve a realistic attitude to breast-feeding. Certainly breast milk is best for the baby, and the warm, nurturing relationship between mother and infant can't be bought in a can, but don't sacrifice yourself entirely to the notion of demand feeding. To my mind, we have gone too far in a reaction against the rigid four-hour feeding schedule of our mothers' day, letting ourselves be slave and martyr to the baby. Unless you genuinely enjoy having the baby with you at all hours of the day and night, derive total pleasure from letting the infant suckle at your breasts any time over a twenty-four-hour period, and are unconcerned by your own lack of sleep and revival periods, I advise you to keep those feedings to a certain limit: every three hours at a maximum.

Having watched women feed on demand, I have to say I do not believe their babies are hungry every hour or half hour. The babies want to suckle, but they can use a pacifier. The babies don't learn to fill their stomachs at one feeding, preferring the ease and comfort of round-the-clock snacks. But they are learning, very early on, to impose on your life, to take over and demand your total attention, instead of blending and fitting in with *your* routine.

If you insist on only giving your baby breast milk, you can express some to refrigerate so your husband can give the baby a bottle of your milk during the night, allowing you precious time to catch up on sleep. If your milk supply begins to wane, it no doubt means you are suffering from lack of sleep and the fatigue of new motherhood that comes from giving away all your resources while not concentrating on restocking the supply. No amount of advice seems to help women once this cycle has set in: whether it be to change her diet, drink more fluids, take brewer's yeast, sip wine to relax her—whatever the latest tips involve. You could try a supplemental bottle of formula given to the baby by someone else during the day or night, so you can sleep. Or, if your doctor will allow it, and the baby is not too young, try a supplement of cereal, which will satisfy the baby's hunger and take some of the pressure off you.

Total breast-feeding does not suit every woman, just as we differ in the types of food we eat, our sex lives, and our choice of just about everything. Just because your friend or sister has fed her baby a particular way does not mean you have to. Always try and keep a perspective on things. You do count, just as much as your baby. If you are overtired, overwrought, and underslept, your baby will not be getting enough milk, and ultimately your crack-up or collapse from exhaustion will be of no use to the baby anyway.

TIME OUT FROM MOTHERHOOD

Stay-at-home mothers and working mothers find themselves equally vulnerable to the permanent-mother trap. All the components of psychological stress we have been discussing in this book, the potential triggers of PPD, are linked to the concept that being a mother can take over your whole life and can overtake you in the process. Whether you feel a resulting loss of self-esteem, confused self-image, or lack of identity and feeling of entrapment, the antidote to the problem is the same: you must find ways of relocating yourself, best achieved by taking some time out for yourself.

Ideally you should be able to work this time out with your husband, for he will be wanting his own private time too, and trade-offs should be possible. You are bound to run into problems with devising time out. One of the running problems of losing your sense of identity is not knowing what you want to, or could do, on your own. Try and keep in touch with some aspects of your former life: whether that means an exercise class, regular running or swimming, dance lessons, or evening classes in the pursuit of photography or macramé; meeting a friend for dinner or an evening at her home; going to a movie with your husband or by yourself; going to a museum; or just blissful time to yourself to browse in the department stores (even if you can't afford to buy anything).

The important part is that this should not be time you guiltily arrange with a sitter and then dash in and out for a frenzied hour or less. You should be able to leave your baby, or children, with someone you trust and take the time you deserve and need.

The problem of not knowing who you are any more, or what you could do that would really free you from motherhood, was faced by Regina V. Although her answer included nothing startling or exotic, the way she reached that conclusion is interesting for any new mother. Robin S. faced a different problem: how to manage time to herself with the stress of full-time work and not enough time anyway.

Regina and Robin: Getting Out on Their Own

Regina and her husband Ronnie had moved to a new neighborhood before having their baby Lesley, and as Regina was back at work three days a week, she had had no time to build up any friendships near their home. Lesley had been sick, and she had had to take days off work to stay with her. It was midwinter, and Regina was cooped up and resentful at being stuck in the house all day and at her husband's relative freedom.

Too much work and responsibility, plus resentment and hostility, led Regina into depression. Three weeks of this mood and Ronnie begged her to find some personal outlet. He was feeling guilty about always being the one to ask for time to go play basketball or do something at the weekend, leaving Regina with all the responsibility, increasingly depressed because she was so trapped. But Regina panicked. What could she do? Her sense of self had gone. Her old formulas didn't apply any more.

Regina finally went to the local library one evening, where she spent two hours away from the baby, the house, and her misery. It may not have seemed wildly exciting, but it was *her* time. "I had a wonderful time doing just as I pleased, and even a year later I still go to the library once a week. Now I get books and toys for Lesley, and read for my own pleasure, and I write in my diary." Regina knew she could rely on those two hours every Wednesday. The time alone helped bring her frazzled nerves together, in what had been a frightening and lonely time.

Robin S., who was back at work full time with a six-month-old baby, also found herself sliding into depression from the lack of time to herself, rest, and recreation. After a year of this routine the crisis came for Robin. "My husband finally yelled at me that I had to see a psychiatrist. I was so angry that I stormed out of the house. As far as I could see it was *his* fault, not mine. But somehow that argument between us helped bring my mind around to a different way of thinking. I realized I had become martyrish. So I arranged to take a week off work and instead of staying home with the baby, I took her to the sitter's and I just spent every day doing what I wanted: long glorious days doing nothing, browsing in stores, going to galleries. I felt guilty, of course, particularly when a male colleague said, 'Are you going to take another week off to spend with your baby? That must have been so nice for you.' "

Finding time to ourselves that is our own, *without guilt,* will be a valuable way of reducing stress and tension and of restoring some of the shattered identity and lowered self-esteem that can be such strong triggers for PPD. It's a question of learning to relax into this new role of motherhood, rather than rushing headlong into its intensity.

DIET AND EXERCISE

So much is written these days on the efficacy of diet and exercise for overcoming virtually every problem that many women assume there must be a particular diet or exercise regimen to avoid or combat PPD. For those with mild depression and a good diet, strenuous exercise will help shift mood and bring about a more cheerful frame of mind in which to review the rest of the picture. If moderate-to-severe depression has set in, it is unlikely to be shifted by these means alone.

There are some tips for developing a diet that can help guard against PPD. First, make sure you eat a good healthy diet. Even if you are trying to lose pregnancy weight, do not go on a crash diet after childbirth, as that will only encourage the onset of depression (from the lack of nutrition that helps stabilize the metabolism under all circumstances). If you are breast-feeding, remember you need to build up your calorie intake, over that of a normal diet, to ensure there is enough caloric energy left over for *you* after the baby has devoured his or hers.

It is advisable to eat little and often in the months after childbirth, every two or three hours, as your body will feel most comfortable with the optimum blood sugar levels. If your starch level becomes low, sugar is removed from the bloodstream by a spurt of adrenalin, and the buildup of adrenalin helps create tension and irritability.

The premenstruum and the postpartum period, according to Katharina Dalton, share a curious factor: in both, the gap between normal and low blood sugar levels narrows. In both crucial times we are more than normally subject to depression.

OTHER DIETARY TIPS INCLUDE:

1. Take multivitamin tablets containing folic acid and vitamin B_6 (pyridoxine). Iron supplement is also helpful.
2. Do not go back on the Pill, even if you are afraid of another pregnancy, for the artificial hormone progestogen will induce depression.
3. Give up caffeine in coffee or sodas, as it increases anxiety and irritability and could help the onset of PPD.
4. Do not take tranquilizers, as they will make you feel sleepier and mask the real symptoms of PPD.
5. Eat foods containing potassium, such as bananas, tomatoes, and oranges, to counter potential potassium loss after birth.

If you are feeling sluggish, with no particular joy in life, you may wonder how anyone could suggest strenuous exercise as a way out of PPD. If only you knew how to find the energy, you think to yourself, that would be half the problem solved. However, if there is any way to make yourself begin running, swimming, or exercising as in aerobic classes, the results may well be very encouraging. Expending energy helps restore depleted energy. And the resulting happy feelings induced by the hormonal changes caused by the exercising will begin to trigger your biochemical system back into balance.

Do not expect any overnight cures. Eventually the advantages of exercise will begin to pay off in more ways than one: first, it will have gotten you out of the house; second, the exercise in itself is a good way of leaving motherhood concerns behind; and third, exercise works on the neuroendocrine balance and releases the neurotransmitters we know are necessary for a happy mood. Exercise, it is believed, releases the endorphins, which are the brain's natural opiates and mood enhancers. Hence the natural high exercisers experience, and the way they become addicted, too.

IS STRENUOUS EXERCISE SAFE AFTER BIRTH?

Can you partake in such active exercise shortly after childbirth? Kate B. had been very involved in sports before having her baby. A karate fanatic, Kate sent me the following information, which, as the material was aimed at women in professional football or softball, would be good advice for any form of exercise.

"Since it takes a lengthy time, roughly six months after delivery, for the muscles and soft tissues of the female body to readjust themselves to the prepregnant state, women should avoid being hit during this time. The muscles are unable to withstand a blow, and so there is a risk of injuring the internal organs. It would appear logical to me that this advice could be expanded to any contact sports; specifically, I am thinking of karate. It seems that physically a woman does not have the needed ability to harden her muscles to protect her inner organs from a blow in the first six months.

"My physical therapist, who was working with me for a broken hand after delivery, cautioned me not to do any ballistic exercises or sports until at least two months after I terminated nursing. He explained that it takes that long for relaxin (the hormone) to leave the body, that if ballistic exercises were persisted in, I would run risk of injuring joints or ligaments, which were still quite loose. So I decided against jogging or jumping rope until that time."

KEEPING YOUR MARRIAGE ALIVE

Marriage has to be worked at harder now than perhaps at any time in the couple's relationship. It is so easy to let that affection, passion, companionship you both shared dissipate, given the all-devouring work and demands of dealing with a new baby or a growing family. As women have so often noted, missing out on that one stable, solid, supportive form of love has quickened their descent into PPD. If you find yourself devoting all your energies and time to the baby; if you realize you are riddled with resentment at your husband's relative freedom and lack of entrapment in his new fatherhood; if you see that your lack of sexuality is caused by the changes in your relationship to him and the growing relationship with the baby; then do stop, take note, talk it over with him, and make some real efforts to stop the downward progress.

However tied you feel to the baby, you must take time for you as a couple. Baby-sitters can be hired to give you both evening time to get out of the house together. Even if socializing seems too much of an effort, going out together for dinner, to the theater, or to a movie, can relieve you of some of that permanent-mother trap that so easily overpowers, even if this is a second or third baby (each new child changes the rules of the preceding game).

Women have described, in desperation, booking a hotel room for the night and inviting their husbands to join them, leaving the baby, if they were lucky, with a grandmother or some other relative. Others have turned to marriage counseling or family therapy in an effort to restore those bonds that once had been so strong and suddenly appear withered and lifeless. One very good method of rejuvenating a marriage—that my husband and I try to fit in once a year—is to go off on a minivacation together, a sort of second honeymoon, without baby or children, and simply enjoy being lazy, relaxed, and loving together again as we once used to be. Some couples will find it harder than others to leave young children behind, even for four days or a long weekend. To them, I offer this advice: think hard about the effects on the children of being so abandoned, by all means, but think too about the effects on your marriage of no time to yourselves, no chance to be lovers again. The children's peace of mind has to be balanced against your relationship with each other. Being divorced, in the end, is certainly not going to help the children.

AVOIDING ISOLATION

Isolation is a dangerous condition during this time of change and transition. It is also a very frequent complaint of new mothers, whether they have decided to stay home with the baby or have returned to work. The stay-at-home mother obviously has to carve out a whole new life; maybe she has left old friends behind in the workplace and knows no one in the neighborhood home during working hours. The working mother may find herself the only person in her workplace, or at her level, with a new baby; maybe she feels alienated from other mothers, who, she imagines, are all real stay-at-home types.

When we become parents, we naturally tend to drift away from or lose touch with old friends, as our needs, demands, and amount of time and energy available all change. Until we have sorted out our new self-image it can be hard to make new friends. What if you don't see yourself as a mother yet? You may struggle to avoid befriending other mothers. What if you fear your own inadequacy as a mother, blaming yourself if your baby is colicky and stressful, and believing that you are a failure? You will likely avoid other mothers' company for fear that they will judge you as harshly as you are judging yourself.

Isolation encourages depression to take root if we bottle up feelings and channel all our emotions onto the baby. Talk on the phone if you cannot find anyone nearby. If you don't believe that any other new mothers or any of your former friends would be sympathetic, seek some form of professional or supportive help.

Very often friends will be found among those very women we have decided are hostile and not sympathetic, like the other new mothers in our neighborhood, who, we are convinced, are going about their transition with not a drop of a difficulty. Just look at all those contented smiles, we torment ourselves. If there is an organized group of new mothers or of both parents, in the area I highly recommend joining one. In a group with regular meetings, the talk just flows, and those together-looking, organized mothers will be admitting just how afraid and lonely they have been. Strong, lasting friendships are often formed and sealed in these very early days of new mothering.

One level of isolation we may not have considered, before becoming a mother, is whether we have a strong supportive background of female friends. Many young women, in loving relationships with their husbands, lost the friendships of school and college days in turning their loyalty over to their husbands. Many women these days work in male-dominated professions or industries and find they meet few women during the work day and have little need of female companionship in the evenings. When they become mothers they may find few women they can turn to for support.

Vicky: No Communication with Mother

One woman you may rediscover as a friend, despite the complexities of the relationship, will be your mother. Vicky M. really had not wanted to have a baby, certainly not at the time of conception. Newly married, happy being a wife, working in the same company as her husband, able to travel with him on his business trips, she was content with life the way it was. When she became pregnant in her late twenties, however, neither Vicky nor Don felt they could abort their child, and so they eagerly awaited the birth. Vicky gave up her job—another woman determined to act out her image of real mother.

Within weeks of Sarah's birth, Vicky found she resented the baby and her new life with a terrible anger. "I lived each day as if I were in mourning for my previous life." Loneliness had set in, with her lost freedom, lost job, lost opportunities to meet with women friends, who were all colleagues in the place of work; lost opportunity to travel with her husband, and a lost closeness with him. Vicky felt very much alone, deserted and, of course, depressed.

When Don was away on a business trip, Vicky was left at home with the baby for three weeks. She knew she was on the verge of cracking up. Finally, she phoned her mother, who lived about an hour and a half's drive away, and with whom, she admitted, she had never been close. Her mother insisted she come to stay while Don was absent. Her younger sister would be home from college and they would be able to help her with Sarah. Vicky had never been the type to open up to her mother or sister, never been one to admit she was in need or that they could help. She was ill at ease discussing her depression, isolation, and resentment. "But," she said, "it was during those two weeks I spent at my mother's house that I began to adapt to my new role a little better. My mother, father, and sister were very helpful with the baby, giving me time to get more rest than I had been used to, baby-sitting so I could go shopping. I spent a lot of time talking with my mother and sister, and although I didn't go as far as to tell them of my feelings of *regret* about having the baby, the conversations and their company were very therapeutic. I suppose my depression began to shift then, though I still don't find it easy."

CHANGING ATTITUDES

Talking to people, finding new friends, working on the relationship with our husbands—all such basic, normal parts of everyday life, yet ironically sometimes so difficult to keep up with once we become parents, and once PPD has begun to set in, depriving us of the energy levels, drive, and commitment we used to hold with confidence and ease. I want to talk now about changing our attitudes toward mothering. This may not come easily without some professional (counseling, psychiatric, or medical) help. But if we can swing our mind round to a new, positive, way of looking at parenting, that can be an enormous help in breaking depression.

We have to turn our mind away from the traditional and socially acceptable standards that have induced in us guilt, fear of inadequacy and failure, and a confused self-image. Try reminding yourself of the following facts in the mornings on waking.

1. We are not alone in our unacceptable feelings. Probably the majority of women are going through similar changes in mood and behavior, and are equally unprepared to meet its challenges.
2. We will feel guilt. Dr. Spock tells us we shouldn't, but it is nearly impossible to rid motherhood of guilt.
3. Help or support is available in different forms, but it may take a lot of digging out. Doctors you are used to relying on may offer not only no help, but no sympathy. It may take strength

and courage to find decent professional care, and that is unfair when we have so little strength or courage at this time.

4. We can own up that being a mother is not as easy as we had expected or fantasized, that we don't like it as much as we had imagined, that we are not perfect mothers or perfect parents, but we're not so bad, either.
5. Losing our independence, freedom, and sense of self, particularly if we have been used to a career, active working life, regular exercise routine, or hobbies, will be difficult whether we stay home full time and yearn for our past varied life or continue working and yearn for past moments of peace and time to ourselves.

Robin: Not Perfect, but a Good Mother and Wife

"I forced myself to repeat every day, especially in the mornings, 'I am not perfect, but I am a good mother and wife.' This eventually led to an attitudinal change, an acceptance of the imperfections of motherhood. I also learned to predict the onset of depression and divert it. I would either warn my husband and we'd talk, or I would permit myself a 'primal scream' if I was alone. Then I'd spend the rest of the day problem solving or accepting the unsolvable," explained Robin S.

Robin came to that change in attitude during her own particular crisis. After nearly a year of depression following the birth of their daughter, Robin's husband suddenly lost all patience. He had tried to persuade her to seek psychiatric help, but Robin had refused. Now he warned her to straighten up or else. His threat made her focus exactly on what was going on. Time had run out, and if she was to continue refusing any outside help she would have to solve her own problems or she would lose husband, dreams, and everything she had always wanted.

Kate: Short-circuiting PPD a Second Time

Some women have sought psychotherapeutic help in a desire to talk over their problems and inner conflicts with a sympathetic, objective person. Kate B. decided to see a women's counselor after her six-month PPD in the hope of finding a solution to this problem should she want a second baby. Kate was a very busy, active woman before motherhood and had suffered from entrapment, resentment of her husband, and other typical PPD symptoms. The counselor gave the following advice, which Kate felt helped change her own attitude.

1. There is no simple solution—women are as individual as their feelings.
2. Feelings are going to come whether they are wanted or not.
3. It helps greatly to ventilate—any way you can do it—whether through yelling, or physical exercise, or talking with someone.
4. There is an element of grieving in every crisis: job loss, PPD, surgery, illness, disease, death. It helps to read up on the subject of loss.
5. Talk. Find a good listener, someone in your same situation or who has been through it.
6. After you figure out how you are feeling, accept those feelings as normal, OK, fine, and not selfish. Then think about what you need to feel better and take some action.
7. Find support groups ahead of time.
8. Don't advise someone else that everything will be fine and let it go at that. That is ignoring the hurt. You need someone to whom you can say, "I hurt," who will acknowledge it and sympathize. You need solutions, rather than denial of the situation.

GETTING THE FEELINGS OUT ON PAPER

As talking is evidently one of the best means of defusing emotional tension, if there is no one to turn to who will listen, if you cannot afford, resent or feel threatened by the idea of seeking professional help, then keeping a journal, pouring out those shameful thoughts on paper, can be an invaluable process. Many women have instinctively tried this device and found that it did help to release the emotions; even better, in a couple of months they could read it back and gain support from the realization that they had changed and developed in that time.

Sharon W. was seeing a therapist for her PPD, but had refused to take a course of antidepressants, wanting to control or come to terms with her moods without drug help.

"I have learned to control PPD to some degree," she said. "When I feel it coming on, instead of getting mad at my elder daughter, I put her in bed and I write in my journal. It's my private book. I write that I can't stand my husband, that I wish I'd never met him. That's not what I really feel, but I need to express my anger and disappointment. Later I comment on those entries when I'm feeling better. I reread it every couple of months."

Regina: Beside Herself with Anger

Regina V., whom we met before, describing how her release from entrapment and the ties of motherhood had finally been discovered in the library, commented that the feelings of resentment and anger she had been bottling up inside her—with no close friend to talk to, with work, baby-sitters, a child's illness, winter claustrophobia, and a host of other problems—found great release when she wrote about them. She kept a diary that was of great help to her. One part of it, during those winter months of crisis, read like this:

"Feb. 18th. Due to this stressful week with Lesley being sick; *me* being sole caretaker; *me* having to miss work and to call in sick to say I wouldn't be in; *me* having to arrange and rearrange a baby-sitter for Lesley so I could work; *me* having to feed her supper and eat alone because Ronnie was working late and playing basketball or racquetball; *me-me-me!!!* By the time Ronnie got home this evening I was beside myself with anger. I talked with him about my feelings later in the evening after Lesley was in bed.

"I feel bad; I feel defeated; I feel worthless; I feel stagnant; I am depressed; I am resentful; I am unhappy with my body; I am unhappy with my eating habits; I have many problems. I was reaching my breaking point this evening when I even felt Ronnie was *not* my partner any more. That scares me. I felt alone and overburdened. I feel unchallenged and overchallenged with Lesley and housekeeping. I want to earn money, I want to be with

Lesley and care for her, I want Ronnie not to have to work so much, I want him to have Lesley to care for alone—me NOT around. I feel isolated being home with Lesley so much. But I *don't* want her with a sitter more. I can't win. . . . I feel defeated. I wish I had more confidence in myself. I wish I had more respect for myself. I am quickly losing any I had. . . ."

That particular entry led to the confrontation with Ronnie and his plea that she find some outlet for *herself;* that he would look after Lesley one evening a week, on a regular basis. Eventually, by taking the time out, Regina said, "Suddenly I regained a sense of self-worth. It was several weeks before I felt in control of my life again but it did return. It is painful to remember this period of time in my life."

FILLING OUT A QUESTIONNAIRE

Many women who received one of my questionnaires when I was researching this book commented that they didn't mind if I never used their material, it had been such a therapeutic exercise to write about what they had felt. So, for anyone with a secret desire to get a whole load off her chest, I reprint the questionnaire here—for your own personal, private use or to share with a close friend or your husband.

I would like to discuss the following topics:

1. When did you suffer the depression, after a first child, second, or subsequent? After each birth, or only once?
2. Had you heard of PPD, or just of the three-day blues? Were you surprised or shocked to be so depressed?
3. Did you seek any help? From a friend, partner, your husband, ob/gyn, pediatrician, a GP, social worker, priest, preschool teacher, therapist, or hospital emergency room? Or no one?
4. Did you come to your own awareness, or was it pointed out by your husband, a partner, friend, your mother or sister?
5. Do you feel guilty about having such a depression, or at your unacceptable and unexpected feelings?

6. Do you find it hard to speak about it to others in general, to a group of other mothers, to your family?
7. Have you felt any of the following: loss of your own identity; loss of self-esteem; fear that your life is over (or wish that it was); trapped; confused over how you relate to motherhood (or fatherhood); new sympathy or contempt for your own mother; despair; disillusionment; anger at your husband, partner, other women, doctors, the baby, its siblings, your mother or sister, society in general; mourning that you can never be the little girl (or boy) again; emotional emptiness; wondering if it was a terrible mistake?
8. Do you believe other mothers feel this way?
9. Are you an adoptive mother, a stepmother, a single mother (or father)?
10. How has your husband or partner responded? With anger or hostility? With sympathy? By withdrawing from you and the baby?
11. Do you think working mothers suffer PPD more or less than full-time mothers?

As an example of the way some women wrote to me, and so you can share in their frankness and honesty, I am reprinting the following reply from Joan R. She is articulate and typical of the women who are becoming mothers today—facing new concerns, new ambivalence, new demands on their lives as mothers. Joan's reply especially moved me.

1. I suffered PPD after experiencing a miscarriage with my first pregnancy and again (a much more severe bout) after the birth of my second child. There was really no time for PPD after the second birth (third pregnancy)! Also, I had "exorcised my demons" by that time. Any crying I did was from sheer fatigue.
2. I had heard of the blues but I was very surprised to have such a violent case after the first birth. The depression after the miscarriage seemed, to me, to be normal under the circumstances.
3. After the miscarriage, I called my ob-gyn. He was very un-

sympathetic to me and suggested that I seek psychiatric help, as my depression was not normal. Therefore, after the birth of my next child, I *wouldn't* call him. The only reason I had stayed with him was because his office was near my job. My mother and a friend, both of whom had experienced PPD, tried to help but I couldn't talk about it with them.

4. My husband was the one to let me know just how much the PPD was affecting me—and him. He was very worried but sympathetic. My depression went on for about three months before he spoke to me about it. It was as if a dam broke loose within me. All the insecurities in me came out. For instance, my father walked out on my mother when I was four months old. Therefore, in my confused and depressed state, I was trying to figure out how I was going to support this child when my husband left me! I'm sure this sounded crazy but my husband was great about it. He reassured me of his love—for me and our son.

   Motherhood, I believe, is a shock at any age and in any circumstance. I was twenty-nine years old when my son (the first birth) arrived. He couldn't have been more wanted. Yet I felt really trapped and frightened about my ability to take care of this child.

5. I felt guilty about the feelings because I should have been so happy, but instead I was on the brink of despair!
6. I did find it hard to verbalize my feelings until my husband brought them out. I'm active in the Childbirth Education Association and when I'm assisting in a class for expectant parents, I always insist that the group be warned of the possibility of PPD. If it should happen to any of them, they at least know that they are not alone. I encourage anyone who needs a listener to call me.
7. I felt a loss of identity. Instead of being just Joan R., I was somebody's *mother*. I thought my life was over because I couldn't see beyond the endless fatigue. There seemed to be no future. I felt so trapped. I thought that I would never be "free" from the responsibilities that went with motherhood. Also, my son was born in January so I couldn't get out of the house much. I didn't think I was cut out to be a mother (a

little late for that!) and I *was* afraid that I had made a terrible mistake.

One good thing that came of all this was that I gained a new respect for my mother. I really think that having a child makes you appreciate your mother.

I was relived to see the word "despair" in the questionnaire. For me, PPD does not mean "postpartum depression" but "postpartum *despair.*" That had to be one of the lowest points of my life. At times, I questioned my sanity, the futility of my life, even my marriage.

I would like to add that after the birth of my second child, I did change ob-gyns. What a difference! When I became pregnant with my daughter, I spoke with the doctor regarding my previous PPD experiences. He was very sympathetic and promised me that if I needed help, he would be there to offer advice and help.

8. Yes, I believe more mothers have PPD—in varying degrees—than are willing to admit it. Having a baby is supposed to be one of the happiest times of your life. Many women don't want to admit that for some of us—as much as we love our babies—it is anything but happy. Instead it is a time for confusion, despair, feeling unloved and unwanted, not to mention feeling like a giant milk bottle if you are nursing.
9. I am a happily married woman (soon to celebrate my fourteenth wedding anniversary) with a really terrific husband.
10. My husband was bewildered and worried but sympathetic. He never withdrew from the baby or me.
11. I don't think there are any differences between working mothers and full-time mothers when it comes to postpartum depression. The severity may be more or less due to knowing you have to go back to work. The prospect of going back to work helped me to see that there was life after baby!

Good luck with your book. I hope that I helped in some small way. Thank you for letting me share my experiences with you. Sometimes it helps just to talk about it.

Joan

P.S. I am the mother of James (age eight) and Carol (age five). I can truthfully say that, if I had it to do over again, I would. My children are two of the greatest things that have ever happened to me.

FINDING A SYMPATHETIC DOCTOR

So often women have complained about the lack of sensitivity, understanding, or sympathy they have received from family doctors, obstetricians, or even psychiatrists to whom they were referred with PPD, that the question is left hanging: how are we to find a good, aware, sympathetic doctor?

In most cases, a woman goes through pregnancy without giving potential PPD a thought. But after childbirth, with the unexplained and unrecognizable feelings swamping her, she begins a desperate search, or perhaps she tries the one doctor she imagines will help, only to be rebuffed, and is left to deal with the problem herself.

Because there is no national or centralized method in the United States of recognizing or diagnosing cases of PPD, there are many gaps in the services new mothers are offered.

MILD SYMPTOMS

Contact a local mothers' support group (see Chapter 15) or call a warm line (see p. 213) for details of a self-help group for new mothers. Either the meetings themselves, with other women, will be sufficient to dispel some of the symptoms, or they might be able to put you in touch with doctors, counselors, or therapists in your area who are most suitable.

MODERATE SYMPTOMS

If PPD has become heavy, if your depression has persisted for more than a few weeks and nothing you have tried will shift it, you might need some professional care, for therapy and treatment with antidepressant medication. Where to find that help will be the same for you as for women with severe symptoms.

SEVERE SYMPTOMS

Symptoms such as the following require good, prompt treatment: a pattern of not being able to sleep or eat; high anxiety level or panic attacks; a feeling of being utterly unable to cope; a sluggish depression that is so deep you cannot get out of bed let alone look after the baby; not being able to bear touching the baby; constant crying that in itself is disruptive to family life; fear about harming the baby; talk of taking your own life; hallucinations, a feeling that you are worthless and all would be better off without you (see Chapter 4).

SEEKING GOOD HELP FOR MODERATE TO SEVERE SYMPTOMS

If your own family doctor or obstetrician seems unsympathetic, you should call your nearest large teaching hospital and find out if their department of obstetrics/gynecology has a psychiatrist attached. Many departments do team up with a psychiatrist who will have experience with PPD. Or, through the resources list in the Appendix of this book, you may discover a highly trained psychosomatic ob/gyn within your area.

You can contact a local mental health clinic for immediate psychiatric care or ask your family doctor to recommend a psychiatrist. As in the cases described earlier, if you feel you are getting nowhere with a particular psychiatrist, do get a second opinion. You deserve good treatment. Unfortunately, with the lack of knowledge even at the professional level, it may be hard to come by.

WHAT IS GOOD CARE FOR PPD?

A sensitive obstetrician should be able to help with incipient PPD by talking honestly with the woman before childbirth and finding time to meet with her and her husband after the baby has been born. Dr. Elisabeth Herz points out that appropriate training for young obstetricians now includes special seminars in

PPD. Such enlightened training is by no means regulation, but at this Washington, D.C., hospital she feels they are making the right moves. "I am trying to get across to the young doctors that they should be aware of certain risk factors in pregnant women and that certain women should be watched more closely."

To Dr. Herz, the risk factors include the mother being older than average and expecting her first baby or having a lengthy interval since her last baby. Her hormonal profile might show that she had menstruated early, had had irregular and painful periods, and was a PMS sufferer. If her pregnancy was unplanned she would be at high risk, and talking with her might reveal ambivalence about motherhood. If she had been infertile for several years; if there is marital tension at home, or she is feeling unloved or unsupported by her husband; if she is separated or single; if she is lacking in support from family or friends, these would also increase the risk of PPD.

Dr. Herz believes that a conflicted relationship with her mother might be reflected in the woman's higher education or professional level; the career woman may have unconsciously rejected the traditional female role because she experiences it as a threat to her identity. She recommends watching for overanxious or very hostile women and those who feel out of control of their lives. Recent stressful life events should be taken into consideration. At very high risk is a woman with a previous PPD, as the recurrence rate given by some authorities is as high as 20 to 30 percent, and Dalton, after a ten-year follow-up study, found the alarming rate of 68 percent.

An aware obstetrician working with pregnant women would be prepared to meet with the high-risk new mother at least two extra times after childbirth: perhaps asking a nurse to call the mother at home about three weeks after she returned home just to chat and see how the mother feels she is getting along. "The sooner we handle incipient problems the better," Herz has said.

If the obstetrician felt the mother needed referral to a psychiatrist, that could be arranged in conjunction with special PPD professionals in the field. Dr. Herz is trained in both obstetrics and psychiatry, and is thus admirably suited to coping with new mother problems in her postpartum office care. Unfortunately, there are only ten or twelve such professionals in the country.

At the first signs of PPD, after the new mother has talked about her adaptation and problems at home and assessed her mood and personality, Dr. Herz can intervene with individual therapy or she may decide the mother needs some form of medication (probably antidepressants) as well.

The sad truth, however, is that most medical and psychiatric training does not carry specific information about PPD. The level of material available, as witnessed by one of the leading textbooks on ob/gyn, is pathetic and most likely to encourage doctors to see these new mothers as crazy ladies.[54]

"Mental illness complicates about 1 in 400–1000 pregnancies. Traditionally, the causes of postpartum psychosis are infectious, toxic, and idiopathic, although it is now apparent that the condition is not a distinct clinical entity and that the underlying problem is the disintegration of personality structure, usually associated with sexual maladjustment, fear, anxiety, and rejection of the pregnancy. A careful inquiry into the patient's history often shows long-standing problems in making social adjustments and in accommodating to the female role."[55]

SCREENING PREGNANT PATIENTS

For the most part, women with mild to moderate cases of PPD do not seek help, in this country. Their recovery comes from waiting the depression out or they might find help in the parent support groups currently flourishing nationwide.

I must put in a word of reluctance about the trend toward psychological screening of pregnant women to detect high-risk cases. There is one article in the PPD literature, by two Canadian doctors, Braverman and Roux, in which a list of nineteen questions is given to pregnant women in their prenatal clinics or doctors' waiting rooms for them to fill out.[56] The questions are as follows:

1. Did you become very depressed or extremely nervous in the period following the birth of your last child?

2. Are you single or separated?
3. Do you have a mother, father, brother, or sister who has been hospitalized for a mental disorder?
4. Do you have a grandmother, grandfather, uncle or aunt who has been hospitalized for a mental disorder?
5. Did you have an unhappy childhood?
6. Do you have marital problems?
7. Was your pregnancy unplanned (accidental)?
8. Can you honestly say at this time that you really do not desire to have a child?
9. Do you have a bad relationship with your mother?
10. Do you have a bad relationship with your father?
11. Do you have serious problems which worry you at present (financial, personal, or other—underline)?
12. Do you feel that your mother was not a good mother?
13. Do you lack confidence in yourself?
14. Is your general health poor in your opinion?
15. Do you more or less regret that you are pregnant?
16. Do you feel that your mother does not love you?
17. Do you see yourself as an immature, dependent individual?
18. Do you often feel that your husband (boyfriend) does not love you?
19. Did your mother, sister, or grandmother tell you that one can be very sick when pregnant?

The results, they felt, showed the value of preventive psychiatry in spotting certain traits as predictors of PPD: personality factors, immaturity, female role rejection, hostility toward the mother and family, past history of mental illness, and heredity.

My own response on reading those questions was first to wonder how valuable a woman's self-assessment would be to such probing questions, and second to imagine the type of replies I would write sitting in my doctor's office. How many women would admit feeling that their husband or boyfriend did not love them? How many would write down, for the doctor to read, that they regret being pregnant? Third, what if you answered no to all the questions, emerging with a healthy score, and later suffered PPD?

THE POSTPARTUM CLINIC

To my mind, the best form of care for reasonably healthy women who might find themselves sufferers of some form of PPD would be provided by the maternity wings of the hospitals where we deliver our babies. A postpartum clinic, within which we would receive some instruction on baby care in the days immediately after delivery, would also offer advice on potential emotional problems once back at home.

The postpartum clinic would be a bright, airy, friendly, cheerful part of the maternity wing, offering playroom or day care facilities for those mothers who need to return for advice or help, bringing older children with them. Attached to the clinic would be a mother and baby unit for those women who have to be readmitted in the year after childbirth for intensive psychiatric treatment.

Women in the maternity wards need not be aware of the psychiatric admissions. Their concerns will revolve around how to care for their baby and what will happen when they are back home. The talks, or discussions, would be in groups of ten new mothers with a nurse, social worker, psychiatrist, and recent mother who can talk about her own experiences. Hormonal shifts and biochemical upheavals would be explained, so all new mothers would know what might happen and, if it did, what they should do to help themselves.

The meetings would offer basic advice and send the mother away with a kit including telephone numbers of people to contact if in doubt, distress, or depression.[57] The telephone numbers would include parent support groups in the community, the hospital social worker, and psychiatrists and therapists who work with PPD mothers. Women might also exchange home numbers for moral support. Finally, they would be advised that they will be welcome back at the postpartum clinic for pediatric advice or motherhood advice any time they want to drop in for coffee and someone to talk to.

Lacking such hospital-provided services, women have been

banding together in an effort to help one another through the crises of parenting (as the crises obviously continue beyond the first year of a baby's life), and the results are found in the burgeoning movement of parent support groups.

Chapter 15

SHARING AND SUPPORT

"Why has it taken so long for a really very simple idea to catch on; that parents should get together for support and help on how to deal with their kids; that they don't have to operate in isolation, fear, and guilt?" said Sandra Rodman Mann, who has set up a masters' program in teaching parent skills at Fordham University in New York. She was speaking at a conference in New York (May 1984) on "Parent Support Groups: Coming of Age in the 80s." The conference was widely attended by staff of many such groups that are opening around the country, by members of family service and mental health agencies, by politicians, activists, and mothers. Workshops were offered, ideas aired and debated, questions raised, contacts made and shared.

After years of the isolation we all experience to some degree with the nuclear family, one of the best ways out of the depths of despair and depression and the gnawing attacks of anxiety is to help one another and ourselves by meeting in organized, nonjudgmental groups of fellow mothers (or parents). Together we can learn about infant and childcare, family skills and management; together we can act as forceful pressure groups in the community and among the professions.

"Somewhere out there in the midwest," said Sandra Rodman Mann, "the Family Resource Coalition has flourished. There is a kind of magic about such great organizations, which are volunteerism at its best." The FRC, the national organization that coalesces these support groups, came into being after a conference in May 1981 and has proved to be a highly successful, determined, outward-reaching body with headquarters in Chicago.

Bernice Weissbourd, president of the coalition and founder of a parent support group in Evanston, Illinois, said very firmly, "We no longer view parents as vehicles for the care of children. We recognize the need for healthy 'parent development' too. Parenthood must be a creative period of self-growth, not a guilt-laden duty."

There were many different types of support groups under discussion at the conference. Family Resource Coalition has put together the most up-to-date list of their organizations and affiliates across the country for this book, which you will find in the resources list in the Appendix. Perhaps this will be the most valuable information for any of us to have at our fingertips: a direct line into sharing and support with other mothers.

PEP: SANTA BARBARA

As was mentioned in Chapter 7, Jane Honikman, of Santa Barbara, California, founded Postpartum Education for Parents (PEP) with three women friends. These women had no example to follow in the early 1970s, when instinct told them they could not be the only young mothers sitting around in the park wondering what had happened to their lives, their marriages, and their sanity, and wondering how they were going to get through this daunting period of life called parenthood. Their belief in the importance of what they were doing led them on through problems of organization, confirmation, support, and funding to become a successful voluntary self-help agency.

"The reality of caring for a totally dependent infant twenty-four hours a day shattered our expectations," Jane explained. "We were learning about our infants and how to care for them through trial and error. (Somehow our babies did not fit the descriptions of the babies in the books.) We had many questions about our feelings and concerns, and believed there had to be someone who knew how to make parenting this precious new being as purely satisfying as we had expected it to be. We felt confused, inadequate, and overwhelmed. In order to maintain the expected aura of joy that new parents 'should' feel, however, we bottled up our continuing sense of panic and kept on smiling."

They intended to set up a parent support group that would offer discussion groups with a format for sharing common concerns and at the same time solve some typical problems. They wanted to offer a twenty-four-hour telephone service—which they called a warm line to offset the negative connotations of hot or help line—for those mothers who may not have had the courage or energy to go out to a meeting at that point in their lives, but who needed to talk to someone, anyone, in moments of despair, panic, or fear.

The women began their operation by contacting various professionals in the area, from the local ob/gyn doctors and hospitals, pediatricians, county mental health services, and the AAUW (American Association of University Women) to whose Goleta Valley branch they applied for a research and project grant that helped with printing costs.

They agreed to work with mothers who volunteered to be facilitators for their group meetings. The volunteers would be trained as active listeners and would also take shifts on the warm line.

PEP is now a wide-ranging service that sends a speaker to each childbirth preparation class to distribute PEP brochures and to talk about their services. They ask parents to sign a Childbirth Class Summary and Postpartum Call Sheet if they wish to have a volunteer contact them after the birth of their baby. Brochures are distributed to local physicians' offices and family centers.

The Santa Barbara PEP is perhaps rare in its outreach efforts. They follow up the childbirth class talk with a postpartum call made when an announcement of the birth appears in a local paper or they learn of a birth from the Lamaze teacher.

The telephone caller informs the mother where and when PEP groups meet in her area (they have evening groups for working mothers or fathers) and asks a simple, concerned question, such as "How has it been going?" Groups endeavor to match the babies' ages as closely as possible, and the facilitators encourage discussion. Usually, talk at first centers on some problem of childcare, then moves on to the mothers' concerns about themselves. The groups of about eight members meet every two to three weeks for two hours or so. Sometimes the women become such good friends they decide to continue meeting as their babies grow older, without the facilitator.

MELD: MINNEAPOLIS

Another such organization is in Minneapolis. Called MELD, it was set up by Ann Ellwood in 1973, in her effort to answer the question of how families can be strengthened. Ellwood felt that parents can learn much from each other, they can give each other support, and they should be free to make informed choices. MELD is also a nonprofit organization, providing group meetings with facilitators and comprehensive material within five subject areas: health, child development, child guidance, family management, and personal growth. There is a MELD for new parents, teenage mothers, parents of preschool or school age children, and bicultural, military, or religious families. The groups meet about eight times, weekly or biweekly.

MELD has been widely expanded over the last ten years, and their programs are now in forty-five different locations across the country. They have replication packages that include training material for the agency, a site coordinator, and volunteer facilitators, and material for parents.

THE MOTHERS' CENTER: NEW YORK

In Nassau County, Long Island, New York, the Mothers' Center Development Project was set up in 1981, run by Lorraine Slepian and Marge Milch. They intend their Mothers' Centers to be as valuable to the community as schools and hospitals—and they wish every community had one. The aim is to provide research and services on mothering, pregnancy, childbirth, and health care. Again, members meet in peer groups, by age of their children, and a separate room is provided for childcare (but one part of their philosophy is that mothers should not mind their child wandering in and out during the group meeting), with two trained facilitators, for a limited number of sessions. Very often, after finishing a ten-week session, the mothers sign up again for another session or perhaps take a break and then return.

The Mothers' Center aims to work with parents throughout the children's stages of development. As Lorraine Slepian says, "Most communities are similar to Nassau County in the inadequate provision of services to pregnant women and mothers. What services there are focus only on the physical aspects of pregnancy. There is little opportunity for women to discuss their deep personal concerns and to find out how to obtain other services they may require." At present there are over twenty Mothers' Centers in other locations.

If you are interested in joining such a group or in helping to set one up, you should contact the Family Resource Coalition in Chicago or any of the local and regional groups in your area (see the resources list in the Appendix). The bigger agencies, such as PEP, MELD, and the Mothers' Center, have manuals and guides that explain how to set up such an organization in your community.

There may also be less formal groups of women meeting that you could track down by contacting one of the national or regional self-help clearing houses (see Appendix). Very often the YWCA, your hospital, or a pediatrician's office will help in getting interested mothers together.

WORKING MOTHERS' GROUPS

Although many of these groups do offer evening sessions for working mothers (or fathers), working women may find such groups scarce out of office hours. Many working mothers are too exhausted even to imagine taking in a parenting group in their spare hours.

One new line of approach is for such groups to be held in the workplace. Before you get too excited about this idea, the only one I know of in existence has been set up by the Financial Women's Association (FWA), which has a Working Mothers Group. Its chairperson, Nan Foster Rubin, is an assistant vice president with Citibank in New York.

When Nan was six months pregnant, a few other women at her level were also pregnant or had young children, and so the idea of a support group was devised. They were all serious professionals who had to cope with problems of childcare, juggling personal and professional lives, and the basic concern of how to be a successful working mother.

The group began in 1979 and has been formally recognized by the FWA. They have a monthly luncheon (in midtown or downtown) to which they invite a visiting speaker or just talk about what is on their minds. It provides support for mothering as well as networking for professional concerns. As Nan notes, "We do talk outside those meetings, too."

The FWA's Working Mothers Group is no doubt the best way to beat that special form of isolation of being the only woman in your company with these concerns. Other professional or union agencies should set up similar groups that are not limited to one company or workplace. However, if you don't have anyone to talk to about your mothering or parenting problems, you might have to be the person who starts a group going. Someone, somewhere, is going to have to find the energy and drive necessary.

EPILOGUE

When I set about writing this book, I thought that most women would be reluctant to discuss the subject of PPD, that I would be forcing my ideas on unwilling listeners. I was surprised and overwhelmed by the abundance of replies that poured in to my request for experiences of the blues or postpartum depression, by the ease with which women spoke, and by the gratitude they expressed at being able to talk and, that someone was finally researching and addressing the issue. PPD is as important and valid a consideration, as much a part of pregnancy and childbirth, as those other topics traditionally discussed in childbirth preparation or Lamaze classes. Yet it is the one area of having a child that we have largely ignored because it is unwelcome, taboo, and certainly does not fit with the generally rosy view we have of motherhood.

I am convinced that honesty, awareness, and understanding of PPD's symptoms, why it happens, and how it can be handled will be as great a liberating force in contemporary women's lives as the struggle to gain the vote, equal rights at work, or sexual emancipation were in the past. We do not have to be tied to the yoke of accepting our mothering in the traditional way it has always been promoted. We do not have to believe that PPD symptoms are evidence of an abnormal reaction. We are complex, rounded, weird, wise; above all we are human, individual women, with needs and desires that have to be satisfied in a variety of ways.

I want to see a different future for my daughters, one in which they not only accept that work is an integral and important part of their lives, but also one in which they view motherhood as an exciting, challenging step into another stage of life, which will help them grow and develop as fully realized people and which, like any stage of growth, won't be a breeze.

If we accept the physical and psychological upheavals women undergo in becoming mothers, I believe we will truly be viewing women as the fascinating, boundlessly creative people they really are.

Appendix

RESOURCES

WHOM CAN YOU GO TO FOR HELP?

If you feel you are in need of a doctor with some specialized knowledge of PPD, whether an obstetrician, psychiatrist, or family doctor, the following list includes those doctors known to have more than average interest or information on PPD's causes and best methods of treatment. (It is an ad hoc compilation from literature and other sources and not verification of the doctor's ability.)

Psychiatrists/Psychologists

ANTON, RAYMOND F., JR, M.D., Dept. of Psychiatry and Behavioral Sciences, Medical University of South Carolina, 170 Ashley Ave., Charleston, S.C. 29401

AUCHINCLOSS, ELIZABETH, M.D., Payne Whitney Clinic, The New York Hospital, 525 E. 68th St., New York, N.Y. 10021

BLACKMAN, LIONEL H., M.D., 2001 Embassy Dr., West Palm Beach, Fla. 33401

BLIX, SUSANNE, M.D., Dept. of Psychiatry, Indiana University School of Medicine, 1100 West Michigan St., Indianapolis, Ind. 46223

BRESSLER, BERNARD, M.D., 104 Berrington Court, Richmond, Va. 23221

BROWN, W. A., M.D., Dept. of Psychiatry, Brown University, Prospect, Providence, R.I. 02904

CAMPBELL, JAN L., M.D., Dept. of Psychiatry, VA Medical Center, 4801 Lynwood, Kansas City, Kan. 64128

CARRANZA, JOSE, M.D., Dept. of Psychiatry, Baylor College of Medicine, Texas Medical Center, Houston, Tex. 77030

EATON, MERRILL T., M.D., 602 S. 45th St., Omaha, Neb. 68106

GERNER, ROBERT H., M.D., UCLA-NPI, 760 Westwood Plaza, Los Angeles, Cal. 90024

GORODETSKY, GALINA, M.D., 3608 Sacramento St., San Francisco, Cal. 94118

HAMILTON, JAMES A., M.D., Ph.D., 2832 Baker St., San Francisco, Cal. 94123

HENDRIE, HUGH C., M.D., Albert E. Stern Prof. and Chairman, Dept. of Psychiatry, Indiana University School of Medicine, 1100 West Michigan St., Indianapolis, Ind. 46223

HERZOG, ALFRED, M.D., Suite 815, 85 Jefferson St., Hartford, Conn. 06106

HITTELMAN, DR. JOAN, Box 12-3, Dept. of Psychiatry, Downstate Medical Center, 450 Clarkson Ave., Brooklyn, N.Y. 11203

JAMISON, DR. KAY R., Affective Disorders Clinic, Dept. of Psychiatry, UCLA School of Medicine, Los Angeles, Cal. 90024

KLEIN, JUDITH, 100 W. 12th St., Apt. 6K, New York, N.Y. 10011 (psychotherapist)

LABRUM, ANTHONY H., M.D., 601 Elmwood Ave. (Box 668), Rochester, N.Y. 14642

LEVIN, MOLLY HALL, M.D., Payne Whitney Clinic, The New York Hospital, 525 E. 68th St., New York, N.Y. 10021

MCCURDY, LAYTON, M.D., Prof. and Chairman, Dept. of Psychiatry and Behavioral Sciences, Medical University of South Carolina, 171 Ashley Ave., Charleston, S.C. 29401

MELGES, FREDERICK T., M.D., 506 E. Forest Hills Blvd., Durham, N.C. 27707

O'HARA, MICHAEL W., Ph.D., Dept. of Psychology, University of Iowa, Iowa City, Iowa 52242

PASNAU, ROBERT O., M.D., UCLA School of Medicine, 760 Westwood Plaza, Los Angeles, Cal. 90024

RAY, LEWIS, M.D., 2429 Ocean Ave., San Francisco, Cal. 94127

SAKS, BONNIE, M.D., 195 Colony Road, New Haven, Conn. 06511

SCHNEIDMAN, BARBARA, M.D., M.P.H., 3846 Cascadia Ave. South, Seattle, Wash. 98118

SHOLITON, MARILYN, M.D., University of Cincinnati College of Medicine, Dept. of Psychiatry, 231 Bethesda Ave., Cincinnati, Ohio 45267

SHRIVASTRVA, RAM, 51 Newport Ave., Tappan, N.Y. 10983

SEBASTIAN, SIMON, M.D., Dept. of Psychiatry, Louisiana State University Medical Center, Box 33932, Shreveport, La. 71130

STEINER, MEIR, M.D., Ph.D., Assoc. Prof. McMaster Psychiatric Unit, St. Joseph's Hospital, 50 Charlton Ave. E., Hamilton, Ontario, Canada L8N 1Y4

TARGUM, STEVEN, M.D., 2033 K St. NW, Washington, D.C. 20006

TRAPNELL, RICHARD H., M.D., 909 Hyde St., San Francisco, Cal. 94109

WILLIAMS, LYNNE H., M.D., East Twelve Fifth, Suite 203, Spokane, Wash. 99202

WINOKUR, PROF. GEORGE, Dept. of Psychiatry, University of Iowa, 500 Newton Road, Iowa City, Iowa 52242

WOODLE, JOANNE, M.D., Dept. of Psychiatry, University Hospital, SUNY at Stonybrook, N.Y. 11794

WOMEN'S PSYCHOTHERAPY REFERRAL SERVICE, INC., 25 Perry St., New York, N.Y. 10014

Psychiatric Obstetricians and Gynecologists

GOOD, RAPHAEL S., M.D., Clinical Prof. of Obstetrics and Psychiatry, University of Texas, University Blvd., Galveston, Tex. 77550

HERZ, ELISABETH K., M.D., Assoc. Prof. for Ob/Gyn and Psychiatry and Behavioral Sciences, Dept. of Ob/Gyn, George Washington University, 2150 Pennsylvania Ave. NW, Washington, D.C. 20037

ROSENTHAL, MIRIAM B., M.D., Asst. Prof. of Psychiatry, Asst. Prof. of Reproductive Biology, Dept. of Obstetrics, Case Western Reserve Medical School, University Circle, Cleveland, Ohio 44106

SMALL, ELIZABETH CHAN, M.D., Assoc. Clinical Prof. of Obstetrics/Gynecology and Psychiatry, Tufts University School of Medicine, Boston, Mass. 02111

Obstetricians

FEINSTEIN, THEODORE A., M.D., 255 S. 17 St., Philadelphia, Pa. 19103

GRAHAM, DAVID, M.D., Dept. of Gynecology/Obstetrics, Johns Hopkins University School of Medicine, 108 Marvey, Baltimore, Md. 21205

LAFERLA, JOHN, M.D., University of Michigan, K2026 Holden, Ann Arbor, Mich. 48109

SCHULMAN, HAROLD, M.D., Chairman, Dept. of Obstetrics and Gynecology, Albert Einstein College of Medicine of Yeshiva University, 1300 Morris Park Ave., New York, N.Y. 10461

SMITH, DENNIS, M.D., Dept. of Obstetrics, Case Western Reserve Medical School, University Circle, Cleveland, Ohio 44106

All Other Doctors and Researchers

BLISS-HOLTZ, V. JANE, 343 Third Ave., Lindenwold, N.J. 08021 (Researcher)

BRADLEY, CHRISTINE, Ph.D., 4775 Chancellor Blvd., Vancouver, B.C., Canada V6T 1C8 (Researcher)

BRAUNSTEIN, GLENN, M.D., Director, Div. of Endocrinology, Cedars-Sinai Medical Center, Schuman Bldg., Room 516, Los Angeles, Cal. 90048 (Endocrinologist)

EZRIN, CALVIN, M.D., 18372 Clark St., Suite 226, Tarzana, Cal. 91356 (Endocrinologist)

KANE, FRANCIS, M.D., 700 Fannin St., Houston, Tex. 77030 (Researcher)

PAFFENBARGER, RALPH, M.D., Dept. of Epidemiology, Stanford University School of Medicine, Stanford, Cal. 94305 (Epidemiology)

PARRY, BARBARA, M.D., Clinical Psychobiology Branch, National Institute of Mental Health, Bethesda, Md. 20857 (Psychobiology)

RASMUSSEN, HOWARD, M.D., Dept. of Internal Medicine, Yale University School of Medicine, 333 Cedar St., New Haven, Conn. 06510 (Medicine)

WEHR, THOMAS, M.D., Clinical Psychobiology Branch, National Institute of Mental Health, Bethesda, Md. 20857 (Psychobiology)

Nursing

AFFONSO, DR. DYANNE, UCSF School of Nursing, Parnassus Ave., San Francisco, Cal. 94122

FAWCETT, JACQUELINE, Ph.D., F.A.A.N., University of Pennsylvania School of Nursing, 420 Service Drive/S2, Philadelphia, Pa. 19104

GERDS, ROBERTA, R.N., M.N., UCLA School of Nursing, Center for Health Sciences, Los Angeles, Cal. 90024

REEDER, SHARON, R.N., Assoc. Prof. UCLA School of Nursing, Center for Health Sciences, Los Angeles, Cal. 90024

YORK, RUTH, Ph.D., B.S.H., University of Pennsylvania School of Nursing, 420 Service Drive/S2, Philadelphia, Pa. 19104.

Professional Organizations

The Marcé Society. For the years 1984 to 1986, the president will be
Channi Kumar, M.D.
Institute of Psychiatry
De Crespigny Park
London SE5 8AF
England.

American Society of Psychosomatic Obstetricians and Gynecologists. The secretary/treasurer at present is
Dennis H. Smith, M.D.
University Hospitals
2105 Adelbert Road
Cleveland, Ohio 44106

PARENT SUPPORT GROUPS

Another line of action in seeking help for PPD is to join a parent support group (or a mothers' group) in your neighborhood. The wonderful organization *Family Resource Coalition* has coordinated all the groups nationwide that are well-organized and members of FRC. If one of the groups mentioned below is in your area, do get in touch. They are all voluntarily run.

Alabama

FAMILY COUNSELING CENTER
6 South Florida St.
Mobile, Ala. 36606
205/471-3466

FAMILY SERVICE DIVISION
FAMILY & CHILD SERVICES
3600 8th Ave., S.
Birmingham, Ala. 35222
205/324-3411

Alaska

FAMILY CONNECTION
1836 W. Northern Lights Blvd.
Anchorage, Alaska 99503
907/279-0551

CENTER FOR CHILDREN & PARENTS
808 East St.
Anchorage, Alaska 99501
907/276-4994

JUNEAU WOMEN'S RESOURCE CENTER
110 Seward St., Room 6
Juneau, Alaska 99801
907/586-2977

Arizona

COMMUNITY INFORMATION & REFERRAL SERVICES, INC.
1515 East Osborne
Phoenix, Ariz. 85014
602/263-8856; 1-800-352-3792

ENRICHMENT FOR PARENTS
655 North Craycroft
Tucson, Ariz. 85711
602/881-0935

NEW PARENT PROGRAM
JEWISH FAMILY SERVICE
102 North Plumer Ave.
Tucson, Ariz. 85719
602/792-3641

Arkansas

THE PARENT CENTER
1501 Maryland
Little Rock, Ark. 72202
501/372-6890

California

APPLE PARENTING CENTER
70 Skyview Terrace
San Rafael, Cal. 94903
415/492-0720

CALIFORNIA PARENTING INSTITUTE
1030 Second St.
Santa Rosa, Cal. 95129

DEPARTMENT OF CHILD DEV./PARENT EDUCATION
LONG BEACH CITY COLLEGE
4901 East Carson St.
Long Beach, Cal. 90808
213/420-4454

FAMILY RESOURCES
P.O. Box 963
Bolinas, Cal. 94924
415/868-0616

PARENT EDUCATION PROGRAMS
SAN FRANCISCO COMMUNITY COLLEGE
1860 Hayes St.
San Francisco, Cal. 94117
415/346-2246

PARENTS PLACE
3272 California St.
San Francisco, Cal. 94118
415/563-1041

CHILDREN'S HEALTH COUNCIL
CHILD REARING EDUCATION AND COUNSELING PROGRAM
100 Willow Road
Palo Alto, Cal. 94304
415/326-5530

PARENT SUPPORT CENTER NETWORK
FAMILY SERVICE AGENCY
817 de la Vina
Santa Barbara, Cal. 93101
805/965-1001

POSTPARTUM EDUCATION FOR PARENTS (PEP)
P.O. Box 6154
Santa Barbara, Cal. 93160
805/964-2009

PRESCHOOL AND INFANT PARENTING SERVICE (PIPS)
THALIANS MENTAL HEALTH CENTER
8730 Alden Dr.
Los Angeles, Cal. 90048
213/855-3500

A PLACE FOR PARENTS, INC.
2019 14th St.
Santa Monica, Cal. 90405
213/452-3823

STEPHEN S. WISE PARENTING CENTER
15500 Stephen S. Wise Dr.
Los Angeles, Cal. 90024
213/476-8561

Colorado

FAMILY SUPPORT SERVICES
601 South Irving
Denver, Colo. 80219
303/935-9510

JEWISH FAMILY & CHILDREN'S SERVICES
300 South Dahlia, #101
Denver, Colo. 80220
303/399-2660

METROPOLITAN STATE COLLEGE
PARENT EDUCATION RESOURCE CENTER
1006 11th St.
Denver, Colo. 80204
303/629-8362

PARENTS PLUS
P.O. Box 7515
Colorado Springs, Colo. 80933
303/471-3238

Connecticut

CHILD CARE COUNCIL OF WESTPORT-WESTON
90 Hillspoint Road
Westport, Conn. 06880
203/226-7007

MOTHERING CENTER, INC.
235 Cognewaugh Road
Cos Cob, Conn. 06807
203/661-1413

PARENTS TOGETHER
48 Maple Ave.
Greenwich, Conn. 06830
203/869-1979

Delaware

FAMILY SERVICE OF DELAWARE
809 Washington St.
Wilmington, Del. 19801
302/654-5303

District of Columbia

FAMILIES & CHILDREN IN TROUBLE (FACT)
FAMILY STRESS SERVICES OF D.C.
1690 36th St., NW
Washington, D.C. 20007
202/965-1900

THE FAMILY PLACE
1848 Columbia Road, NW
Washington, D.C. 20009
202/265-0149

Florida

FAMILY CENTER OF NOVA UNIVERSITY
3301 College Ave.
Fort Lauderdale, Fla. 33314
305/475-7471

PARENT EDUCATION PROJECT
VALENCIA COMMUNITY COLLEGE
P.O. Box 3028
Orlando, Fla. 32802
305/299-5000

PARENTING PROJECT
PEACE RIVER CENTER
1745 U.S. Highway 17 South
Bartow, Fla. 33830
813/533-3141

PARENT RESOURCE CENTER
42 East Jackson St.
Orlando, Fla. 32802
305/425-3663

Georgia

THE MOTHERS' CENTER OF ATHENS
190 Lavender Rd.
Athens, Ga. 30606
404/549-4640

THE MOTHERS' CENTER OF ROME
Route 1, 313 Haywood Valley
Armuchee, Ga. 30105
404/291-9914

CHILD SERVICE & FAMILY COUNSELING CENTER
1105 West Peachtree, NE
Atlanta, Ga. 30357

Hawaii

HAWAII FAMILY STRESS CENTER
KAPIOLANI CHILDREN'S MEDICAL CENTER
1317 Punahou St.
Honolulu, Hawaii 96826
808/947-8634

Illinois

BEVERLY FAMILY CENTER
9300 S. Pleasant St.
Chicago, Ill. 60620
312/779-1230

EARLY YEARS PROGRAM
ORCHARD MENTAL HEALTH CENTER
8600 Gross Point Road
Skokie, Ill. 60077
312/967-7300

FAMILY CENTER
229 South Bench St.
Galena, Ill. 61036
815/777-1560, 777-2348

FAMILY FOCUS
2300 Green Bay Road
Evanston, Ill. 60201
312/869-4700

PARENT/CHILD NETWORK
P.O. Box 784
Tinley Park, Ill. 60477
312/795-1949

MOMS, INC.
P.O. Box 59229
Chicago, Ill. 60659
312/583-7997

PARENTS & CHILDBIRTH EDUCATION SOCIETY (PACES)
P.O. Box 213
Western Springs, Ill. 60558
312/964-2048

NORTHSIDE PARENTS' NETWORK
P.O. Box 10584
Chicago, Ill. 60610
312/871-0453, 477-2839

PARENTS & CHILDREN TOGETHER (PACT)
405 Wagner Road
Northfield, Ill. 60093
312/446-5370, 251-4451

PARENTAL STRESS SERVICES
59 East Van Buren, #1618
Chicago, Ill. 60605
312/427-1161

PARENTHESIS
405 South Euclid
Oak Park, Ill. 60302
312/848-2227

PARENT SUPPORT NETWORK
5600 South Woodlawn
Chicago, Ill. 60637
312/288-2353, 241-5164

ROGERS PARK FAMILY NETWORK
1545 West Morse
Chicago, Ill. 60626
312/743-2818

VIRGINIA FRANK CHILD DEVELOPMENT CENTER
3033 West Touhy
Chicago, Ill. 60645
312/761-4550

FAMILY SERVICE CENTER OF SANGAMON COUNTY
1308 S. 7th St.
Springfield, Ill. 62703
217/528-8406

Indiana

CATHOLIC CHARITIES BUREAU
603 Court Building
Evansville, Ind. 47708
812/423-5456

FAMILY HOUSE, INC.
203 Franklin
Valparaiso, Ind. 46383
219/464-4160

PARENTS HELPING PARENTS
3410 West Virginia St.
Evansville, Ind. 47712
812/479-8423, 425-5525

PARENTS TOGETHER
PORTER COUNTY FAMILY SERVICES
2588-P Portage Mall
Portage, Ind. 46386
219/762-7181

PARENT–YOUNG CHILD PROGRAM
Family & Child Studies
Dept. of Home Economics
Ball State University
Muncie, Ind. 47306
317/896-5018

FAMILY FOCUS OF WHITLEY COUNTY
P.O. Box 497
Columbia City, Ind. 46725
219/691-2297

Iowa

THE PEOPLE PLACE
120 South Hazel
Ames, Iowa 50010
515/233-1677

FAMILY RESOURCE CENTER
2530 University Ave.
Waterloo, Iowa 50701
319/235-6271

FAMILY & CHILDREN'S SERVICE OF DAVENPORT
115 W. 6th St.
Davenport, Iowa 52803
319/323-1852

Kansas

McPHERSON FAMILY LIFE CENTER
Box 1252
McPherson, Kans. 67460
316/241-6603

FAMILY & CHILDREN'S SERVICE
5424 State St.
Kansas City, Kans. 66102
913/287-1300

Kentucky

PARENTS' PLACE
201 Mechanic St.
Lexington, Ky. 40507
606/233-0444

FAMILY & CHILDREN'S AGENCY
1115 Garvin Place
Louisville, Ky. 40201
502/583-1741

Louisiana

FAMILY TREE PARENTING CENTER
P.O. Box 31233
Lafayette, La. 70503
318/988-1136

PARENTING CENTER
7343-C Florida Blvd.
Baton Rouge, La. 70806
504/924-0123

PARENTING CENTER
200 Henry Clay Ave.
New Orleans, La. 70018
504/895-3574

Maine

LINCOLN COUNTY PARENT RESOURCE CENTER
P.O. Box 966
Damariscotta, Maine 04543
207/563-1938

COMMUNITY COUNSELING CENTER
622 Congress St.
Portland, Maine 04101
207/774-5727

Maryland

PARENT CONNECTION
4701 Sangamore Road
Bethesda, Md. 20816
301/320-2321

PARENT EDUCATION RESOURCE CENTER
12518 Greenly Dr.
Silver Springs, Md. 20906
301/871-3873

FAMILY LIFE CENTER, INC.
10451 Twin Rivers Road
Columbia, Md. 21044
301/997-3557

Massachusetts

THE PARENT CONNECTION
700 Grove St.
Worcester, Mass. 01605
617/852-5658

COPING WITH THE OVERALL PREGNANCY & PARENTING EXPERIENCE (COPE)
37 Clarendon St.
Boston, Mass. 02116
617/357-5588

THE PARENT CONNECTION
1210 Massachusetts Ave.
Arlington, Mass. 02174
617/641-2229

THE MOTHER CONNECTION
P.O. Box 59
Andover, Mass. 01810
617/470-0539

THE PARENTS CENTER OF HOPKINTON
ST. PAUL'S EPISCOPAL CHURCH
Wood Street
Hopkinton, Mass. 01748
617/435-3062

Michigan

THE CHILD & FAMILY NEIGHBORHOOD PROGRAM
33577 Berville Court
Westland, Mich. 48184
313/729-2610

FAMILY SERVICE ASSN. OF DETROIT & WAYNE COUNTIES
51 West Warren
Detroit, Mich. 48201
313/833-3733

FAMILY GROWTH CENTER
215 North Capitol
Lansing, Mich. 48933
517/371-4350

MOTHER HAVEN
Haslett Professional Building
5681 Shaw St.
Lansing, Mich. 48909
517/339-8691

PARENTS SUPPORTING PARENTS
700 Fuller N.E.
Grand Rapids, Mich. 49503
616/247-1373

NEIGHBORHOOD FAMILY RESOURCE CENTER OF THE CENTER FOR URBAN STUDIES
WAYNE STATE UNIVERSITY
5229 Cass Ave.
Detroit, Mich. 48202
313/577-2208

Minnesota

MINNESOTA EARLY LEARNING DESIGN (MELD)
123 East Grant St.
Minneapolis, Minn. 55403
612/870-4478

PARENTING RESOURCE CENTER
P.O. Box 505
Austin, Minn. 55912
507/437-7746

RURAL FAMILY DEVELOPMENT
STAPLES PUBLIC SCHOOLS
422 2nd St.
Staples, Minn. 56479
218/894-2430

Mississippi

FAMILY SERVICE ASSN. OF GREATER JACKSON
1510 N. State St.
Jackson, Miss. 39202
601/353-3891

Missouri

THE FAMILY CENTER—A GROWING PLACE
7423 Wellington
Clayton, Mo. 63105
314/726-1666

FAMILY & CHILDREN SERVICES OF KANSAS CITY
THE LIVING CENTER FOR FAMILY ENRICHMENT
3515 Broadway
Kansas City, Mo. 64111
816/753-5325

JEWISH COMMUNITY CENTERS ASSN.
PRIME TIME PROGRAM
2 Millstone Dr.
St. Louis, Mo. 63146
314/432-5700

EARLY EDUCATION PROGRAMS
FERGUSON-FLORISSANT SCHOOLS
655 January Ave.
Ferguson, Mo. 63135
314/595-2355

LADUE EARLY CHILDHOOD CENTER
10601 Clayton Road
St. Louis, Mo. 63131
314/993-5724

THE MOTHERS' CENTER OF ST. LOUIS
516 Loughborough
St. Louis, Mo. 63111
314/353-1558

Nebraska

FAMILY SERVICE ASSN. OF LINCOLN
1133 H St.
Lincoln, Nebr. 68508
402/476-3327

FAMILY SERVICE
2240 Landon Court
Omaha, Nebr. 68102
402/345-9118

NEWBORN AND PARENT SUPPORT GROUP
421 N. Lincoln
Hastings, Nebr. 68901
402/462-5515

New Hampshire

THE CHILDREN'S PLACE—A FAMILY RESOURCE CENTER
P.O. Box 576
Concord, N.H. 03301
603/224-9920

New Jersey

NEW JERSEY SELF-HELP CLEARINGHOUSE
ST. CLARE'S HOSPITAL
Pocono Road
Denville, N.J. 07834
1-800/452-9790

FAMILY COUNSELING SERVICES
10 Banta Place
Hackensack, N.J. 07601
201/342-9200

THE TEANECK PARENTS CENTER
61 Church St.
Teaneck, N.J. 07666
201/836-8271

FAMILY LIFE RESOURCES
203 2nd St.
Fanwood, N.J. 07023
201/889-4270

New Mexico

THE PARENTCRAFT PROGRAM
P.O. Box 6852
Albuquerque, N.M. 87197
505/256-1191

New York

FAMILIES FIRST
250 Baltic St.
Brooklyn, N.Y. 11201
718/855-3131

FAMILY DYNAMICS, INC.
225 Park Avenue South, #734
New York, N.Y. 10003
212/260-4344

THE MOTHERS' CENTER DEVELOPMENT PROJECT
129 Jackson St.
Hempstead, N.Y. 11550
516/486-6614; toll free from outside N.Y. 800-645-3828 (call for location of ten Mothers' Centers in New York)

THE PARENT CENTER
MT. KISCO ELEMENTARY SCHOOL
West Hyatt Ave.
Mt. Kisco, N.Y. 10549
914/666-8215

PARENTING CENTER
92nd STREET YM-YWHA
1395 Lexington Ave.
New York, N.Y. 10028
212/427-6000, x206

THE PARENTING PLACE
METROPOLITAN HOSPITAL CENTER
Pediatrics Dept.
1901 1st Ave.
New York, N.Y. 10029
212/360-7329

PARENT RESOURCE CENTER
FLOWER HILL SCHOOL
Campus Dr.
Port Washington, N.Y. 11050
516/883-4000, x230, 231

PARENTS' PLACE, INC.
3 Carhart Ave.
White Plains, N.Y. 10605
914/948-5187

PARENTING EDUCATION PROGRAM (PEP) OF BROOKLYN
P.O. Box 49, Downstate Medical Center
450 Clarkson Ave.
Brooklyn, N.Y. 11203
718/270-2176

WEBSTER AVENUE FAMILY RESOURCE CENTER
134 Webster Ave.
Rochester, N.Y. 14609
716/654-8673

North Carolina

FAMILY & CHILDREN'S SERVICE
301 S. Brevard St.
Charlotte, N.C. 28202
704/332-9034

FAMILY SERVICE OF WAKE COUNTY
3803 Computer Dr.
Raleigh, N.C. 27609
919/781-9317

Ohio

THE FAMILY PLACE
JEWISH COMMUNITY CENTER
3505 Mayfield Road
Cleveland Heights, Ohio 44118
216/382-4000, x218, 282

FOCUS ON MOTHERS
NORTHEASTERN YWCA
5257 Montgomery Road
Cincinnati, Ohio 45212
513/351-6550

MOTHERS' CENTER OF CINCINNATI
776 Hanson Dr.
Cincinnati, Ohio 45240
513/851-5963

HEIGHTS PARENT CENTER
13263 Cedar Road
Cleveland Heights, Ohio 44118
216/321-0079

WHOLE PARENT/WHOLE CHILD
76 Bell St.
Chagrin Falls, Ohio 44022
216/247-6920

Oklahoma

PARENTS' ASSISTANCE CENTER
707 N.W. 8th
Oklahoma City, Okla. 73102
405/232-8227 or 8226

TULSA COALITION FOR PARENTING
1430 South Boulder
Tulsa, Okla. 74119
918/585-5551

Oregon

BIRTH-TO-THREE
1432 Orchard, #4
Eugene, Oreg. 97407
503/484-4401

METROPOLITAN FAMILY SERVICE
2281 N.W. Everett St.
Portland, Oreg. 97210
503/228-7238

Pennsylvania

PARENTING DEPARTMENT
BOOTH MATERNITY CENTER
6051 Overbrook Ave.
Philadelphia, Pa. 19131
215/878-7800, x651

FAMILY SUPPORT CENTER
2 Baily Road
Yeadon, Pa. 19050
215/622-5660

PARENT RESOURCE ASSN.
P.O. Box 2111
Jenkintown, Pa. 19046
215/576-7961

BRIGHT BEGINNINGS WARM LINE
MAGEE WOMEN'S HOSPITAL
Forbes Halket
Pittsburgh, Pa. 15213
412/647-4546

Rhode Island

WOONSOCKET FAMILY CENTER
460 S. Main St.
Woonsocket, R.I. 02895
401/766-0900

South Carolina

FAMILY SERVICE OF CHARLESTON COUNTY
Community Services Building
30 Lockwood Blvd.
Charleston, S.C. 29401
803/723-4566

South Dakota

FAMILY SERVICE
1728 South Cliff Ave.
Sioux Falls, S.D. 57105
605/336-1974

POSITIVE PARENT NETWORK
P.O. Box 2792
Rapid City, S.D. 57709
605/348-9276

Tennessee

FAMILY SERVICE OF MEMPHIS
2400 Poplar Bldg.
Memphis, Tenn. 38112
901/324-3637

Texas

AVANCE
1226 N.W. 18th St.
San Antonio, Tex. 78207
512/734-7924

DALLAS ASSN. FOR PARENT EDUCATION
13551 N. Central Exp. #12
Dallas, Tex. 75243
214/699-0420

FAMILY SERVICE CENTER
2128 Avenue P
Galveston, Tex. 77550
409/762-8636

FAMILY RESOURCE CENTER
3203 Nacogdoches Road
San Antonio, Tex. 78217
512/657-3094

HOUSTON ORGANIZATION FOR PARENT EDUCATION
3311 Richmond, #330
Houston, Tex. 77098
713/524-3089

Utah

FAMILY SUPPORT CENTER
2020 Lake St.
Salt Lake City, Utah 84105
801/487-7778

DAVIS COUNTY SCHOOL DISTRICT
PARENT EDUCATION RESOURCE CENTER
100 South 200 East
Monte Vista Center
Farmington, Utah 84025
801/451-5071

Vermont

FRANKLIN COUNTY FAMILY CENTER
86 North Main
St. Albans, Vt. 05478

LAMOILLE FAMILY CENTER
Box 274
Morrisville, Vt. 05661
802/888-5229

Virginia

FAMILY SERVICE, INC.
116 West Jefferson St.
Charlottesville, Va. 22901
804/296-4118

Washington

FAMILY SERVICES OF KING COUNTY
107 Cherry St., #500
Seattle, Wash. 98104
206/447-3883

PARENT COOPERATIVE FAMILY EDUCATION PROGRAM
COMMUNITY COLLEGE OF SPOKANE
Institute of Extended Learning
W. 3305 Ft. Wright Dr., MS 3090
Spokane, Wash. 99204
509/459-3737

THE PARENT PLACE
1608 N.E. 150th St.
Seattle, Wash. 98155
206/364-9933, 364-7274

FAMILY LIFE EDUCATION PROGRAMS
PENINSULA COMMUNITY COLLEGE
1502 East Lauridsen Blvd.
Port Angeles, Wash. 98362
206/452-9277

Wisconsin

FAMILY SERVICE OF MILWAUKEE
2819 W. Highland Blvd.
Milwaukee, Wis. 53208
414/342-4558

FAMILY SERVICE OF BELOIT
423 Bluff
Beloit, Wis. 53571
608/365-1244

FAMILY ENHANCEMENT
605 Spruce St.
Madison, Wis. 53715
608/256-3890

MILWAUKEE AREA TECHNICAL COLLEGE
FAMILY LIVING EDUCATION
1015 N. 6th St.
Milwaukee, Wis. 53203
414/278-6835, 278-6219

MILWAUKEE MELD
4385 Green Bay Ave.
Milwaukee, Wis. 53209
414/263-2044

FRC itself can be contacted for any further information; to join the coalition as a member and receive its three-times-a-year *Report*, dues are $15 a year for an individual and $30 a year for an organization. Write to Family Resource Coalition, 230 N. Michigan Ave., Suite 1625, Chicago, Ill. 60601 (312-726-4750).

For any mother wishing to take her interest in parent support groups or parent education further, you might be interested in a degree specialization that has been set up (in 1984) at Fordham University in parent education. Chairperson, Division of Curriculum and Teaching, Room 1102A, Fordham University Graduate

School of Education at Lincoln Center, 113 W. 62nd St., New York, N.Y. 10023.

SELF-HELP CLEARINGHOUSES

If you still have a problem finding a group of parents or mothers in your area, you could try these self-help clearinghouses. The list is furnished by the FRC *Report* (October–December 1983).

SAN FRANCISCO SELF-HELP CLEARINGHOUSE
Mental Health Assn. of San Francisco
2398 Pine St.
San Francisco, Cal. 94115
415-921-4401
Sharon George, Director

CALIFORNIA SELF-HELP RESOURCE CENTER
University of California
Psychology Dept.
405 Hilgard Ave.
Los Angeles, Cal. 90024
213-825-3552
Dr. Douglas Anglin

SAN DIEGO SELF-HELP CLEARINGHOUSE
P.O. Box 86246
San Diego, Cal. 92138
619-275-2344
Ellen Murphy, Director

CONNECTICUT SELF-HELP MUTUAL SUPPORT NETWORK
19 Howe St.
New Haven, Conn. 16511
800-842-1501 or 203-789-7645
Vicki Smith

HILLSBOROUGH COUNTY SELF-HELP CLEARINGHOUSE
Florida Mental Health Institute
13301 N. 30th St.
Tampa, Fla. 33612
813-974-4672
Michelle Kunkel, Coordinator

SELF-HELP CENTER
1600 Dodge Ave., S112
Evanston, Ill. 60201
312-328-0470
Leonard Borman, Director

BERRIEN COUNTY SELF-HELP CLEARINGHOUSE
Riverwood Community Mental Health Center
2681 Morton Ave.
St. Joseph, Mich. 49085
616-983-7781
Rob Hess/Charles Livingston

MINNESOTA MUTUAL HELP RESOURCE CENTER
Wilder Foundation Community Care Unit
919 Lafond Ave.
St. Paul, Minn. 55104
612-642-4060
Thomas Duke, Director

SELF-HELP INFORMATION SERVICES
1601 Euclid Ave.
Lincoln, Nebr. 68502
402-476-9668
Barbara Fox, Director

NEW JERSEY SELF-HELP CLEARINGHOUSE
St. Clare's Hospital CMHC
Denville, N.J. 07834
201-625-6395
Edward J. Madara, Director

BROOKLYN SELF-HELP CLEARINGHOUSE
Heights Hills Mental Health Service
30 Third Ave.
Brooklyn, N.Y. 11217
718-834-7341
Carol Berkvist, Director

LONG ISLAND SELF-HELP CLEARINGHOUSE
New York Institute of Technology
Commack College Center
6350 Jericho Turnpike
Commack, N.Y. 11725
516-499-8800
Robert Slotnick/Abe Jaeger, Co-Directors

NEW YORK CITY SELF-HELP CLEARINGHOUSE
City University of New York
Graduate Center, 1225
33 W. 42nd St.
New York, N.Y. 10036
212-852-4290
Carol Eisman/Fran Dory, Co-Directors

WESTCHESTER SELF-HELP CLEARINGHOUSE
Westchester Community College
Academic Arts Building
75 Grasslands Road
Valhalla, N.Y. 10595
914-347-3620
Leslie Borck, Director

INFORMATION AND REFERRAL SERVICES
United Way of The Columbia Wilamette
718 W. Burnside
Portland, Oreg. 97209
503-222-5555
Nancy Webb-Ranken

PHILADELPHIA SELF-HELP CLEARINGHOUSE
John F. Kennedy CMHC
112 N. Broad St.
Philadelphia, Pa. 19102
215-568-0860, x276
Jared Hermalin, Director

SELF-HELP INFORMATION & NETWORKING EXCHANGE
Voluntary Action Center of NE Pennsylvania
200 Adams St.
Scranton, Pa. 18503
717-347-5616
Arlene Hopkins, Director

DALLAS SELF-HELP CLEARINGHOUSE
Mental Health Assn. of Dallas County
2500 Maple Ave.
Dallas, Tex. 75201-1998
214-748-1998
Carol Madison, Director

GREATER WASHINGTON SELF-HELP COALITION
(Washington, D.C., N. Va., and S. Md.)
Mental Health Assn. of Northern Virginia
100 N. Washington St.
Falls Church, Va. 22046
703-536-4100
Linda Figuerosa, Coord.

National

NATIONAL SELF-HELP CLEARINGHOUSE
CUNY Graduate Center, 1206A
33 W. 42nd St.
New York, N.Y. 10036
212-840-1259
Frank Riessman/Alan Gartner, Co-Directors

MISCELLANEOUS

Working Mothers

Catalyst, 14 E. 60th St., New York, N.Y. 10022 (212-759-9700) is a national organization that tries to help communication between corporations and women in an attempt to resolve career and family issues. They have a book list that might be of help or interest, and a library that is open to the public, full of resources on women, work, and family.

The Conference Board (New York only) is a clearinghouse of information on work and family. The Financial Women's Association Working Mothers Group: contact Nan Foster Rubin through the FWA of New York, 35 E. 72nd St., New York, N.Y. 10021.

Adoptive children

Center of Adoptive Families, 67 Irving Place, New York, N.Y. 10003 (212-420-8811) offers family therapy, advice, support, and help with adoption agencies.

Single Parents

Single Parent Resource Center, 225 Park Ave. S., New York, N.Y. 10003 (212-475-4401) is a clearinghouse for groups of single parents, publishes its newsletter *Speak Out*, and offers advice, support, help with housing, and contact with other single parents.

Parents Without Partners, 7910 Woodmont Ave., Washington, D.C. 20014.

Multiples

Mothers of Twins Club, 5402 Amberwood Lane, Rockville, Md. 20853 (301-460-9108).

Publications

Birthwrites, published by the Houston Organization for Parent Education, Inc., 3311 Richmond Ave., Suite 330, Houston, Tex. 77098. The newsletter of HOPE reaches 4,000 couples in the area.

Practical Parenting, ed. Vicki Lansky. Write for her newsletter to 18326B Minnetonka Blvd., Deephaven, Minn. 55391 (612-475-1505).

Working Parents' Forum, an eight-page bimonthly national newsletter designed to put working parents in touch with the latest information on balancing family and career. It is edited by Pattie Carroll Kearns, R.N., a childbirth and parent educator. Write to Center for Family and Community Education, Inc., P.O. Box 4505, New Windsor, N.Y. 12550 (allow six to eight weeks for delivery).

ICEA Review, a publication of the International Childbirth Education Association, P.O. Box 20048, Minneapolis, Minn. 55420-0048.

NOTES

[1] Dr. Elisabeth Herz, Associate Professor for Gynecology and Obstetrics and Psychiatry, Director of Psychosomatic Ob/Gyn Program at George Washington University Medical Center, 2150 Pennsylvania Ave., NW, Washington, D.C. 20037. For information about other psychosomatic ob/gyns in the country, contact the ASPOG, Secretary-Treasurer, Dr. Dennis H. Smith, University Hospitals, 2105 Adelbert Road, Cleveland, Ohio 44106.

[2] Dr. Katharina Dalton, of London, has published widely on PMS, oral contraceptives, migraine, and puerperal disorders. A list of her articles may be obtained from her office, 100 Harley St., London W.1. The most recent and interesting of her books are *Premenstrual Syndrome and Progesterone Therapy,* 2nd ed. (Chicago: Year Book, 1983); *Once a Month*, 2nd ed. (Claremont, Calif.: Hunter House, 1983); and *Depression After Childbirth* (London: Oxford University Press, 1980).

[3] Dr. James Hamilton, formerly a clinical psychiatrist at Stanford University, California, has been involved in work on PPD for more years than perhaps any other doctor in the United States. For many years he has run a sort of mail-order service as distraught new parents have somehow come across his name, in library catalogues or occasional articles that have reached the public eye, and consequently sought his advice. For two years he acted as secretary of the Marcé Society, retiring from that position in 1984, though he will no doubt continue to remain active in Marcé's cause.

[4] Dr. E. A. Strecker was a well-known practicing psychiatrist in the 1940s, chairman of the psychiatry department at the University of Pennsylvania, consultant to the Surgeons General of the Army and Navy, and adviser to the Secretary of War. In his Foreward to the book *Their Mothers' Sons* (New York: Longmans, 1946), with the subtitle *The Psychiatrist Examines an American Problem,* Eugene Meyer, Chairman of the National Committee on Mental Hygiene, commented

that to Strecker the cold hard facts were that 1,825,000 men were rejected for military service because of psychiatric disorders.

On April 27, 1945, Strecker delivered a lecture before several hundred medical students and physicians at Bellevue Hospital in New York. The lecture has since been controversially titled "the moms lecture" and was influential as the first in a memorial lectureship at the bequest of Dr. Menas Gregory, professor of psychiatry at New York University and head of the psychiatric division at Bellevue. Strecker called his lecture "Psychiatry Speaks to Democracy," but, writes Meyer, it could have been called "Psychiatry Speaks to the Neurotic Moms of Psychoneurotics," for the darts of his comments were directed at the apron-stringing mothers of America and at their indirect effect on democracy. Strecker indicted the doting mother for her sins of commission and omission against her children and, therefore, the nation.

5. Terra Ziporyn, "Rip van Winkle Period Ends for Puerperal Psychiatric Problems," Medical News, *JAMA* 251 (April 1984).

6. The first Marcé Society conference was held in London. This biennial meeting was hosted in San Francisco in 1984, and there is talk of the 1986 conference being held in Edinburgh. The American conference was sadly underrepresented by U.S. doctors and psychiatrists, but everyone is hoping that situation will be rectified by 1986.

7. I. Yalom, D. Lunde, R. Moos, and D. Hamburg, "Postpartum Blues Syndrome," *Archives of General Psychiatry* 18 (1968): 16–27.

8. Two articles so far report unsuccessful attempts to associate specific hormonal changes with mental disorders: P. N. Nott, M. Franklin, C. Armitage, and M. G. Gelder, "Hormonal Changes and Mood in the Puerperium," *British Journal of Psychiatry* 128 (1976); 379–83, and R. Treadway, F. Kane, A. Jarrahi-Zadeh, and M. Lipton, "A Psychoendocrine Study of Pregnancy and the Puerperium," *American Journal of Psychiatry* 125 (1968–69): 1380–86. Very little research has been completed in this fascinating field.

9. I refer readers to two volumes for further help in understanding the psychoendocrine factor: Maggie Scarf's splendid book that so lucidly explains science to the layperson—*Unfinished Business: Pressure Points in the Lives of Women* (Garden City, N.Y.: Doubleday, 1980); and the NIMH booklet, *Depression, Manic-Depressive Illness and Biological Rhythms*, by Eunice Corfman, Science Reports 1 (ADM) 79-889, 1982.

10. Penny Budoff, *No More Menstrual Cramps and Other Good News* (New York: Putnam, 1980).

11. Dane Prugh, *The Psychosocial Aspects of Pediatrics* (Philadelphia: Lea & Febiger, 1982).

12. James Hamilton, M.D., *Postpartum Psychiatric Problems* (St. Louis: Mosby, 1962).

13. "Postpartum Psychiatric Problems and Thyroid Dysfunctions," by Nobuyuki Amino, Osaka University Medical School, Osaka; and "Clinicoendocrine Studies of Postpartum Psychoses," by Nomura, Okano, Harada, Kitayama, Inoue, Yamaguchi, and Hatotani, Mie University School of Medicine, Tsu, Mie. See Proceedings of the Marcé Society Conference, San Francisco, 1984 (for details apply to the Marcé Society secretary).

14. "The Use of Corticoids in Postpartum Psychiatric Illness." See Proceedings of the San Francisco Conference, ibid.

[15] The following information about tranquilizers and antidepressants is taken from *Ms* magazine, May 1984.

"Drugs that calm without impairing consciousness are called tranquilizers. The major ones, used to treat serious cases, such as mania or schizophrenia, are called anti-psychotics (Thorazine, Stelazine, Mellaril, Navane, Prolixin). Minor ones used to treat anxiety and tension are called anti-anxiety drugs such as Valium and Librium. Drugs used to treat depression are anti-depressants, such as Nardil and Elavil" (from *The Doctors and Patients Handbook of Medicines and Drugs* [New York: Knopf, 1984]).

[16] George Winokur, *Depression: The Facts* (New York: Oxford University Press, 1981).

[17] The mother and baby unit at the Massachusetts Mental Health Center is described by Ian Brockington and Frank Margison, "Psychiatric Mother and Baby Units," in *Motherhood and Mental Illness*, ed. Ian Brockington and R. Kumar (New York: Grune & Stratton, 1982). American experience of admitting babies with their mentally sick mothers is described at length in a book by H. Grunebaum, J. Weiss, B. Cohler, C. Hartman, and D. Galland entitled *Mentally Ill Mothers and Their Children* (Chicago: University of Chicago Press, 1975), pp. 223–38.

[18] Ibid.

[19] Mother-baby relationships in psychiatric disorder, as witnessed in the mother and baby unit at the Royal Infirmary, Swinton Grove, Manchester, England, were described by Dr. Frank Margison of the department of psychiatry, a very concerned doctor who has been working with the unit for many years now, at the Marcé Conferences of 1982 and 1984 (see Proceedings of both conferences). Margison is now secretary and bulletin editor of the Marcé Society.

[20] Brockington and Margison, "Psychiatric Mother and Baby Units."

[21] Gregory Zilboorg, "Clinical Issues of Postpartum Psychopathological Reactions," *American Journal of Obstetrics and Gynecology* 73 (1957): 305.

[22] Benjamin Spock, *The Problems of Parents* (Boston: Houghton Mifflin, 1978), pp. 32–38.

[23] Benjamin Spock and Michael Rothenberg, *Dr. Spock's Baby and Child Care* (New York: Pocket Books, 1985), pp. 21–33.

[24] Ibid., p. 29.

[25] Alan Guttmacher, *Pregnancy, Birth and Family Planning* (originally published 1937, revised and updated in 1973 by Viking), p. 272.

[26] Boston Women's Health Book Collective, *Our Bodies, Our Selves* (New York: Simon & Schuster, 1984), and Elizabeth Bing and Libby Colman, *Having a Baby After 30* (New York: Bantam, 1980).

[27] M. Klaus and J. Kennell, *Maternal-Infant Bonding* (St. Louis: Mosby, 1976). This book has now become a classic on the bonding issue, and has proven very helpful in making obstetricians and pediatricians more aware of mothers' and infants' mutual need for early bonding.

[28] Marc Weissbluth, *Crybabies* (New York: Arbor House, 1984) is a convenient paperback that deals thoroughly with the subject of colic in a down-to-earth and sensible fashion.

[29] Ibid., p. 168.

[30] R. Kumar and K. Robson, "Previous Induced Abortion and Ante-natal Depression in Primiparae: Preliminary Report of a Survey of Mental Health in Pregnancy," *Psychological Medicine* 8 (1978): 711–15.

[31] My comments on abortions and their relevance to PPD are my own feelings and should not be imputed to Drs. Kumar and Robson. I would further hate to give the implication that I do not believe in the liberal administration of therapeutic abortions. Given my own feelings about the difficulties of parenting a much-wanted baby, I would never, ever, try to force women to go through with carrying an unwanted pregnancy to term. I do, however, feel we have become too flippant in our use of the procedure and that most women would be grateful for the opportunity to talk about their confused feelings at such a time.

[32] The Women's Psychotherapy Referral Service, 25 Perry St., New York, N.Y. 10014 (212-242-8597), founded in 1972 to provide professional psychotherapists for men and women, comprises over fifty nonsexist therapists in private practice throughout New York City. The service offers to match the client with a therapist who best meets her needs. The initial phone call to the service helps them assess whom to refer you to for an immediate consultation. The initial interview helps the placement process. The New York office may be able to put out-of-town women in search of a good therapist in contact with someone in their area. Judith Klein, who helped with much of the material for this book, was referred to me for this research by the service, as she is known to specialize in women with young children.

[33] George Brown and Tirril Harris, *The Social Origins of Depression: A Study of Psychiatric Disorder in Women* (New York: Free Press, 1978).

[34] PEP has produced three books that may be of interest to mothers, or to those interested in setting up a parents' group (or mothers' discussion group). They also describe the operation of warm lines and the various outreach services that they provide. The books, published in 1978, are *A Guide for Establishing a Parent Support Program in Your Community, A Leader's Guide for Training Volunteers in Parent Support Services,* and *A Volunteer's Reference Guide.* For details of cost, etc., contact PEP (Postpartum Education for Parents), 5049 University Drive, Santa Barbara, Calif. 93111 (805-964-2009).

[35] E. James Anthony and Therese Benedek, eds., *Parenthood: Its Psychology and Psychopathology* (Boston: Little, Brown, 1970). Therese Benedek was a renowned analyst from the Chicago Institute for Psychoanalysis, whose writings on mothering, fathering, the family, and parenthood are well worth reading.

[36] For books on parenting today, I recommend the following: Ellen Galinsky, *Between Generations: The Six Stages of Parenthood* (New York: Times Books, 1981), in which she explores our development as parents through the years of a child's life; S. Jaffe and J. Viertel, *Becoming Parents: Preparing for the Emotional Changes of First-Time Parenthood* (New York: Atheneum 1980); R. Friedland and C. Kort, *The Mother's Book* (Boston: Houghton Mifflin 1981); Howard Osofsky and Joy Osofsky, *Answers for New Parents* (New York: Walker 1980); R. Plutzik and M. Laghi, *The Private Life of Parents* (New York: Dodd, Mead 1983); R. Wolfson and V. DeLuca, *Couples with Children: What Happens to Your Marriage After Baby Comes Home?* (New York: Dembner 1981); and J. Procaccini and M. Kiefaber, *Parent Burn-Out* (Garden City, N.Y.: Doubleday, 1983).

[37] Germaine Greer's latest book, *Sex and Destiny: The Politics of Human Fertility* (New York: Harper & Row, 1984), has a fascinating argument about abstinence and the pressure we come under in the Western world for continuous sexual activity.

[38] "Psychotherapy with Pregnant Women," by Joan Raphael-Leff, in B. Blum,

ed., *Psychological Aspects of Pregnancy, Birthing and Bonding* (New York: Human Sciences Press 1980).

[39] Bob Greene, *Good Morning, Merry Sunshine* (New York: Atheneum, 1984): a father's account of his reactions to the first year of his baby's life.

[40] There are many interesting fatherhood projects being offered these days: for updated information contact the Family Resources Coalition, 230 North Michigan Avenue, Suite 1625, Chicago, Ill. 60601, for information about *Fatherhood USA,* the first national guide to programs, services, and resources for and about fathers (348 pages, $14.95). Started in 1981, with support from several foundations, the Fatherhood Project of Bank Street College, New York, is a national research and demonstration endeavor designed to encourage wider options for men's involvement in child-rearing. The Project is also preparing another book, *The Future of Fatherhood,* a "state of the nation" report on fatherhood and social change, and two manuals based on its demonstration programs: "How to Start a Father-Child Group" and "How to Start a Baby Care Program for Boys and Girls."

[41] Jessie Bernard, *The Future of Marriage* (New York: World, 1972); *The Future of Motherhood* (New York: Dial Press, 1975); *Women, Wives, Mothers: Values and Options* (Chicago: Aldine, 1975).

[42] Lois Gilman, *The Adoption Resource Book* (New York: Harper & Row, 1984).

[43] For articles on adoption, see V. Bental, "Psychic Mechanisms of the Adoptive Mother in Connection with Adoption," *The Israel Annals of Psychiatry* (1965): 24–34; M. Schechter, "About Adoptive Parents," in E. Anthony and T. Benedek, eds., *Parenthood: Its Psychology and Psychopathology* (Boston: Little, Brown, 1970).

[44] J. Selby, L. Calhoun, A. Vogel, and H. E. King, *Psychology and Human Reproduction* (New York: Free Press, 1980). Essays on psychological changes in pregnancy, psychological factors in postpartum reactions, psychological dimensions in controlling conception, and the psychology of the menopause; see particularly pages 87–112 for the section on postpartum reactions.

[45] Frederick Melges, "Postpartum psychiatric syndromes," *Psychosomatic Medicine* 30 (1968): 95–108.

[46] T. Benedek, "Mothering and Nurturing," in Anthony and Benedek, *Parenthood,* pp. 153–66.

[47] H. Blum, "Reconstruction in a Case of Postpartum Depression," *The Psychoanalytic Study of the Child* 33 (1978): 335–61.

[48] To comprehend the seriousness of past treatment of women with mental problems, read Gloria Steinem's very moving account of her mother's mental illness in "Ruth's Song (for She Could Not Sing It)," which is a chapter in her book *Outrageous Acts and Everyday Rebellions* (New York: Holt, Rinehart & Winston, 1983), pp. 129–46.

[49] C. Tetlow, "Psychosis of Childbearing," *Journal of Mental Science* 101 (1955): 629–39.

[50] See Anna Freud, "The Concept of the Rejecting Mother," in Anthony and Benedek, *Parenthood,* pp. 376–86.

[51] Gregory Zilboorg, "The clinical issues of postpartum psychopathological reactions," *American Journal of Obstetrics and Gynecology* 73 (1957): 305.

[52] Spock and Rothenberg, *Dr. Spock's Baby and Child Care;* see "The Parent's Part," pp. 21–33.

[53] Anita Shreve, "The Working Mother as Role Model," New York *Times Magazine,* September 9, 1984, Section 6, pp. 39–45.

[54] David Danforth, ed., *Obstetrics and Gynecology* (New York: Harper & Row 1977): this is the major ob/gyn textbook for medical students.

[55] Danforth, "Psychiatric Disorder," in *Obstetrics and Gynecology,* pp. 449–50.

[56] J. Braverman and J. F. Roux, "Screening for Patients at Risk for Postpartum Depression," *Obstetrics and Gynecology* 52 (1978): 731–36.

[57] Shirley Dick, a clinical social worker at the Memorial Hospital, South Bend, Indiana, has developed a presentation on postpartum emotional adjustments that is used in the hospital's maternity ward. She talks to the new mothers about their unrealistic expectations of handling it all and how the superwoman trap can lead to exhaustion and depression. See her article "New Parenthood Initiation," *Mothers Today,* January–February 1983, p. 12.

BIBLIOGRAPHY

BOOKS

BING, E. and COLMAN, L. *Having a Baby After 30.* New York: Bantam, 1980.

Boston Women's Health Book Collective. *The New Our Bodies, Ourselves.* New York: Simon & Schuster, 1984.

Boston Women's Health Book Collective. *Ourselves and Our Children.* New York: Random House, 1978.

BROCKINGTON, I. F., and KUMAR, R., eds. *Motherhood and Mental Illness.* New York: Grune & Stratton, 1982.

BROWN, G., and HARRIS, T. *The Social Origins of Depression:* A Study of Psychiatric Disorders in Women. New York: Free Press, 1978.

BUDOFF, PENNY. *No More Menstrual Cramps and Other Good News.* New York: Putnam, 1980.

CHODOROW, NANCY. *The Reproduction of Mothering: Psychoanalysis and the Sociology of Gender.* Berkeley: University of California Press, 1978.

COLE, K. C. *What Only a Mother Can Tell You About Having a Baby.* Garden City, N.Y.: Doubleday, 1980.

DALTON, KATHARINA. *Depression After Childbirth: How to Recognize and Treat Postnatal Illness.* London: Oxford University Press, 1980.

DANFORTH, DAVID, ed. *Obstetrics and Gynecology.* New York: Harper & Row, 1977.

FRIEDLAND R., and KORT, C. *The Mother's Book: Shared Experiences.* Boston: Houghton Mifflin, 1981.

GALINSKY, ELLEN. *Between Generations: The Six Stages of Parenthood.* New York: Times Books, 1981.

GREENE, BOB. *Good Morning, Merry Sunshine.* New York: Atheneum, 1984.

HAMILTON, JAMES. *Postpartum Psychiatric Problems.* St. Louis: Mosby, 1962.

JAFFE, S., and VIERTEL, J. *Becoming Parents: Preparing for the Emotional Changes of First-Time Parenthood.* New York: Atheneum, 1980.

KLAUS, M., and KENNELL, J. *Maternal-Infant Bonding.* St. Louis: Mosby, 1976.

KITZINGER, SHEILA. *Women as Mothers: How They See Themselves in Different Cultures.* New York: Random House, 1980.

LICHTENDORF, SUSAN. *Eve's Journey: The Physical Experience of Being Female.* New York: Berkley, 1983.

LYNCH-FRASER, DIANE. *The Complete Postpartum Guide.* New York: Harper & Row, 1983.

MARCÉ, LOUIS VICTOR. *Traité de la Folie des Femmes Enceintes, des Nouvelles Accouchées et des Nourrices.* Paris: J. B. Baillière et Fils, 1858.

NOTMAN, M., and NADELSON, C., eds., *The Woman Patient: Medical and Psychological Interfaces.* Vol. 1. *Sexual and Reproductive Aspects of Women's Health Care.* (New York: Plenum Press, 1978), pp. 73–86 and 107–22.

OAKLEY, ANN. *Becoming a Mother.* New York: Schocken, 1980.

OAKLEY, ANN. *Women Confined: Towards a Sociology of Childbirth.* New York: Schocken, 1980.

OSOFSKY, HOWARD, and OSOFSKY, JOY. *Answers for New Parents.* New York: Walker, 1980.

PASKOWICZ, PATRICIA. *Absentee Mothers.* New York: Universe, 1982.

PLUTZIK, R., and LAGHI, M. *The Private Life of Parents.* New York: Dodd, Mead, 1983.

PROCACCINI, J., and KIEFABER, M. *Parent Burnout.* Garden City, N.Y.: Doubleday, 1983.

PRUGH, DANE. *The Psychosocial Aspects of Pediatrics.* Philadelphia: Lea & Febiger, 1982.

SANDLER, MERTON. *Mental Illness in Pregnancy and the Puerperium.* London: Oxford University Press, 1978.

SCARF, MAGGIE. *Unfinished Business: Pressure Points in the Lives of Women.* Garden City, N.Y.: Doubleday, 1980.

SELBY, J., CALHOUN, L., VOGEL, A., and KING, H. E., *Psychology and Human Reproduction.* New York: Free Press, 1980.

SHEEHY, GAIL. *Passages.* New York: Bantam, 1977.

SPOCK, BENJAMIN, and ROTHENBERG, MICHAEL. *Dr. Spock's Baby and Child Care.* New York: Pocket Books, 1985.

SPOCK, BENJAMIN. *The Problems of Parents.* Boston: Houghton Mifflin, 1978.

WEISSBLUTH, MARC. *Crybabies: Coping with Colic, What to Do When Baby Won't Stop Crying.* New York: Arbor House, 1984.

WELBURN, VIVIENNE. *Post-Natal Depression.* London: Fontana, 1980.

WINOKUR, GEORGE. *Depression: The Facts.* New York: Oxford University Press, 1981.

WOLFSON, R. M., and DELUCA, V. *Couples with Children: What Happens to Your Marriage After Baby Comes Home?* New York: Dembner, 1981.

ARTICLES

ASCH, S., and RUBIN, L. "Postpartum Reactions: Some Unrecognized Variations." *American Journal of Psychiatry* 131 (1974): 870–74.

BARGLOW, P. "Postpartum Mental Illness: Detection and Treatment." In Davis, ed., *Gynecology and Obstetrics,* Vol. 1, Part 2, Chap. 57, pp. 1–11 (1977).

BENEDEK, T. "The Psychobiology of Pregnancy," "Motherhood and Nurturing," and "Parenthood and the Life Cycle." In E. Anthony and T. Benedek, eds., *Parenthood: Its Psychology and Psychopathology.* Boston: Little, Brown, 1970, pp. 137–54, 153–66, 185–208.

BENTAL, V. "Psychic Mechanisms of the Adoptive Mother in Connection with Adoption." *The Israel Annals of Psychiatry* 3 (1965): 24–34.

BLUM, B. "Psychological Aspects of Pregnancy, Birthing, and Bonding." In Barbara Blum, ed., *New Directions in Psychotherapy Series,* Vol. 4. New York: Human Sciences Press, 1980.

BLUM, H. "Reconstruction in a Case of Postpartum Depression." *The Psychoanalytic Study of the Child* 33 (1978): 335–61.

BRAVERMAN, J., and ROUX, J. F. "Screening for Patients at Risk for Postpartum Depression." *Obstetrics and Gynecology* 52 (1978): 731–36.

COGAN, R., ed. "Postpartum Depression," *ICEA Review*, 4 (August 1980): 1–8; from International Childbirth Association, Inc., P.O. Box 20048, Minneapolis, Minn. 55420 (available at a cost of $1.50 per back issue, plus $1 postage and handling).

CORMAN, E. "Depression, Manic-Depressive Illness, and Biological Rhythms." NIMH publication, Science Reports 1, (ADM) 79-889, 1982.

DANIELS, R., and LESSOW, H. "Severe Postpartum Reactions." *Psychosomatics* 5 (1964): 21–26.

FREUD, ANNA. "The Concept of the Rejecting Mother." In E. J. Anthony and T. Benedek, eds. *Parenthood: Its Psychology and Psychopathology.* Boston: Little, Brown, 1970, pp. 376–86.

GARVEY, M. and TOLLEFSON, G. "Postpartum Depression." *Journal of Reproductive Medicine* 39 February 1984: 113–16.

GORDON, R., KAPOSTINS, E., and GORDON, K. "Factors in Postpartum Emotional Adjustment." *Obstetrics and Gynecology* 25 (1965): 158–66.

HAMILTON, JAMES A. "Puerperal Psychoses." In Davis, ed., *Gynecology and Obstetrics* Vol. 2, Part 2, Chap. 24n., pp. 1–11 (1970).

KUMAR, R., and ROBSON, K. "Previous Induced Abortion and Ante-natal Depression in Primiparae: Preliminary Report of a Survey of Mental Health in Pregnancy." *Psychological Medicine* 8 (1978): 711–15.

MCKAY, S., ed. "Maternal Stress and Pregnancy Outcome." *ICEA Review* 4 (April 1980): 1–8.

MELGES, F. "Postpartum Psychiatric Syndromes." *Psychosomatic Medicine* 30 (1968): 95–108.

NOTT, P. N., FRANKLIN, M., ARMITAGE, C., and GELDER, M. G. "Hormonal Changes and Mood in the Puerperium." *British Journal of Psychiatry* 128 (1976): 379–83.

PAYKEL, E. S., EMMS, E., FLETCHER, J., and RASSABY, E. S. "Life Events and Social Support in Puerperal Depression." *British Journal of Psychiatry* 136 (1980): 339–46.

RAPHAEL-LEFF, JOAN. "Psychotherapy with Pregnant Women." In B. Blum, ed., *Psychological Aspects of Pregnancy, Birthing and Bonding.* New York: Human Sciences Press, 1980.

ROSENWALD, G., and STONEHILL, M. "Early and Late Postpartum Illness." *Psychosomatic Medicine* 34 (1972): 129–38.

ROTH, N. "The Mental Content of Puerperal Psychoses." *American Journal of Psychotherapy* 29 (1975): 204–11.

SCHECHTER, M. "About Adoptive Parents." In E. J. Anthony and T.

Benedek, eds., *Parenthood: Its Psychology and Psychopathology.* Boston: Little, Brown, 1970.

SHREVE, ANITA. "The Working Mother as Role Model." New York *Times Magazine,* September 9, 1984, Section 6, pp. 39–45.

TETLOW, C. "Psychosis of Childbearing." *Journal of Mental Science* 101 (1955): 629–39.

TOWNE, R., and AFTERMAN, J. "Psychosis in Males Related to Parenthood." *Bulletin of the Menninger Foundation* 19 (1954): 19–26.

TREADWAY, R., KANE, F., JARRAHI-ZADEH, A., LIPTON, M. "A Psychoendocrine Study of Pregnancy and the Puerperium." *American Journal of Psychiatry* 125 (1968–69): 1380–86.

WAINWRIGHT, W. "Fatherhood as a Precipitant of Mental Illness." *American Journal of Psychiatry* 123 (1966): 4044.

YALOM, I., LUNDE, D., MOOS, R., and HAMBURG, D. "Postpartum Blues Syndrome." *Archives of General Psychiatry* 18 (1968): 16–27.

ZILBOORG, GREGORY. "Clinical Issues of Postpartum Psychopathological Reactions." *American Journal of Obstetrics and Gynecology* 73 (1957): 305.

Index

A

B

C

D

G

H

I

Z